T0259148

Spinal Tumors

Editor

CARLOS H. TORRES

NEUROIMAGING CLINICS
OF NORTH AMERICA

www.neuroimaging.theclinics.com

Consulting Editor
SURESH K. MUKHERJI

August 2023 • Volume 33 • Number 3

ELSEVIER

1600 John F. Kennedy Boulevard • Suite 1800 • Philadelphia, Pennsylvania, 19103-2899

http://www.neuroimaging.theclinics.com

NEUROIMAGING CLINICS OF NORTH AMERICA Volume 33, Number 3
August 2023 ISSN 1052-5149, ISBN 13: 978-0-323-93867-9

Editor: John Vassallo (j.vassallo@elsevier.com)
Developmental Editor: Karen Justine S. Dino

Neuroimaging Clinics of North America (ISSN 1052-5149) is published quarterly by Elsevier Inc., 360 Park Avenue South, New York, NY 10010-1710. Months of issue are February, May, August, and November. Business and editorial offices: 1600 John F. Kennedy Blvd., Suite 1800, Philadelphia, PA 19103-2899. Business and editorial offices: 6277 Sea Harbor Drive, Orlando, FL 32887-4800. Periodicals postage paid at New York, NY, and additional mailing offices. Subscription prices are USD 413 per year for US individuals, USD 745 per year for US institutions, USD 100 per year for US students and residents, USD 483 per year for Canadian individuals, USD 949 per year for Canadian institutions, USD 562 per year for international individuals, USD 949 per year for international institutions, USD 100 per year for Canadian students and residents and USD 260 per year for foreign students and residents. To receive student/resident rate, orders must be accompanied by name of affiliated institution, date of term, and the *signature* of program/residency coordinator on institution letterhead. Orders will be billed at individual rate until proof of status is received. Foreign air speed delivery is included in all *Clinics* subscription prices. All prices are subject to change without notice. POSTMASTER: Send address changes to *Neuroimaging Clinics of North America*, Elsevier Health Sciences Division, Subscription **Customer Service, 3251 Riverport Lane, Maryland Heights, MO 63043. Telephone: 1-800-654-2452 (U.S. and Canada); 314-447-8871 (outside U.S. and Canada). Fax: 314-447-8029. E-mail: journalscustomerservice-usa@elsevier.com (for print support); journals onlinesupport-usa@elsevier.com (for online support).**

Reprints. For copies of 100 or more of articles in this publication, please contact the Commercial Reprints Department, Elsevier Inc., 360 Park Avenue South, New York, NY 10010-1710. Tel.: 212-633-3874; Fax: 212-633-3820; E-mail: reprints@elsevier.com.

Neuroimaging Clinics of North America is covered by *Excerpta Medical/EMBASE,* the RSNA Index of Imaging Literature, *MEDLINE/PubMed (Index Medicus),* MEDLINE/MEDLARS, SciSearch, Research Alert, and Neuroscience Citation Index.

PROGRAM OBJECTIVE

The goal of *Neuroimaging Clinics of North America* is to keep practicing radiologists and radiology residents up to date with current clinical practice in radiology by providing timely articles reviewing the state of the art in patient care.

TARGET AUDIENCE

Practicing radiologists, radiology residents, and other healthcare professionals who utilize neuroimaging findings to provide patient care.

LEARNING OBJECTIVES

Upon completion of this activity, participants will be able to:
1. Review the preferred method for evaluation, imaging characteristics, and key clinical features of spinal cord tumors.
2. Discuss the diagnostic approaches and treatments of pediatric spinal metastases.
3. Recognize other critical modalities used to provide an accurate diagnosis for entities with nonspecific imaging features.

ACCREDITATION

The Elsevier Office of Continuing Medical Education (EOCME) is accredited by the Accreditation Council for Continuing Medical Education (ACCME) to provide continuing medical education for physicians.

The EOCME designates this journal-based CME activity for a maximum of 10 *AMA PRA Category 1 Credit*(s)™.Physicians should claim only the credit commensurate with the extent of their participation in the activity.

All other healthcare professionals requesting continuing education credit for this enduring material will be issued a certificate of participation.

DISCLOSURE OF CONFLICTS OF INTEREST

The EOCME assesses conflict of interest with its instructors, faculty, planners, and other individuals who are in a position to control the content of CME activities. All relevant conflicts of interest that are identified are thoroughly vetted by EOCME for fair balance, scientific objectivity, and patient care recommendations. EOCME is committed to providing its learners with CME activities that promote improvements or quality in healthcare and not a specific proprietary business or a commercial interest.

The planning committee, staff, authors, and editors listed below have identified no financial relationships or relationships to products or devices they or their spouse/life partner have with commercial interest related to the content of this CME activity:

Amit Aggarwal, MD; Mahmud Mossa Basha, MD; Mauricio Castillo, MD, FACR; J. Levi Chazen, MD; Michelle J. Clarke, MD; Juan Pablo Cruz, MD; David J. Daniels, MD, PhD; Amish Doshi, MD; Wende N. Gibbs, MD, MA; Angela Guarnizo, MD; Mai-Lan Ho, MD; Andrei I. Holodny, MD; Matthew T. Houdek, MD; Jack W. Jennings, MD, PhD; S. Mohammed Karim, MD; Sasan Karimi, MD; Majid A. Khan, MD; Kothainayaki Kulanthaivelu, BCA, MBA; Michelle Littlejohn; Kassie McCullagh, MD; Jonathan M. Morris, MD; Kambiz Nael, MD; Luis Nunez, MD; Puneet Pawha, MD; Kyung K. Peck, PhD; Paulo Puac-Polanco, MD, MSc; Roy Riascos, MD; Francisco Rivas Rodriguez, MD; Andres Rodriguez, MD; Peter S. Rose, MD; Atin Saha, MD, MS; Karen Salzman, MD; Michael Schecht, MD; Lubdha M. Shah, MD, MS; David Timaran-Montenegro, MD, MSc; Anderanik Tomasian, MD; Carlos H. Torres, MD, FRCPC, FCAR; Adam Wentworth, MS; Sema Yildiz, MD; Carlos Zamora, MD, PhD

UNAPPROVED/OFF-LABEL USE DISCLOSURE

The EOCME requires CME faculty to disclose to the participants:
1. When products or procedures being discussed are off-label, unlabelled, experimental, and/or investigational (not US Food and Drug Administration [FDA] approved); and
2. Any limitations on the information presented, such as data that are preliminary or that represent ongoing research, interim analyses, and/or unsupported opinions. Faculty may discuss information about pharmaceutical agents that is outside of FDA-approved labelling. This information is intended solely for CME and is not intended to promote off-label use of these medications. If you have any questions, contact the medical affairs department of the manufacturer for the most recent prescribing information.

TO ENROLL

To enroll in the *Neuroimaging Clinics of North America* Continuing Medical Education program, call customer service at 1-800-654-2452 or sign up online at http://www.theclinics.com/home/cme. The CME program is available to subscribers for an additional annual fee of USD 254.00.

METHOD OF PARTICIPATION

In order to claim credit, participants must complete the following:
1. Complete enrolment as indicated above.
2. Read the activity.

3. Complete the CME Test and Evaluation. Participants must achieve a score of 70% on the test. All CME Tests and Evaluations must be completed online.

CME INQUIRIES/SPECIAL NEEDS

For all CME inquiries or special needs, please contact elsevierCME@elsevier.com.

NEUROIMAGING CLINICS OF NORTH AMERICA

SERIES OF RELATED INTEREST

Advances in Clinical Radiology
Available at: Advancesinclinicalradiology.com
MRI Clinics of North America
Available at: MRI.theclinics.com
PET Clinics
Available at: https://www.pet.theclinics.com/
Radiologic Clinics of North America
Available at: Radiologic.theclinics.com

THE CLINICS ARE AVAILABLE ONLINE!
Access your subscription at:
www.theclinics.com

NEUROIMAGING CLINICS OF NORTH AMERICA

Contributors

CONSULTING EDITOR

SURESH K. MUKHERJI, MD, MBA, FACR
Clinical Professor of Radiology and Radiation
Oncology, University of Illinois, Peoria, Illinois,
USA; Robert Wood Johnson Medical School,
Rutgers University, New Brunswick, New

Jersey, USA; Faculty, Otolaryngology–Head
Neck Surgery, Michigan State University,
Farmington Hills, Michigan, USA; National
Director of Head and Neck Radiology, ProScan
Imaging, Carmel, Indiana, USA

EDITOR

CARLOS H. TORRES, MD, FRCPC, FCAR
Professor of Radiology, Department of
Radiology, Radiation Oncology and Medical
Physics, University of Ottawa, Ottawa, Ontario,
Canada

AUTHORS

AMIT AGGARWAL, MD
Assistant Professor, Division of
Neuroradiology, Department of Radiology,
Icahn School of Medicine at Mount Sinai
Hospital, New York, New York, USA

MAHMUD MOSSA BASHA, MD
Professor, Department of Radiology, University
of Washington School of Medicine, Seattle,
Washington, USA

MAURICIO CASTILLO, MD, FACR
Professor, Division of Neuroradiology,
Department of Radiology, The University of
North Carolina at Chapel Hill, Chapel Hill,
North Carolina, USA

J. LEVI CHAZEN, MD
Hospital for Special Surgery, New York,
New York, USA

MICHELLE J. CLARKE, MD
Department of Neurosurgery, Mayo Clinic,
Rochester, Minnesota, USA

JUAN PABLO CRUZ, MD
Assistant Professor of Radiology, Servicio de
Neurorradiología Diagnóstica y Terapéutica,
Instituto de Neurocirugía Dr. Asenjo, Santiago,
Chile

DAVID J. DANIELS, MD, PhD
Department of Neurosurgery, Mayo Clinic,
Rochester, Minnesota, USA

AMISH DOSHI, MD
Associate Professor, Division of
Neuroradiology, Department of Radiology,
Icahn School of Medicine at Mount Sinai
Hospital, New York, New York, USA

WENDE N. GIBBS, MD, MA
Director of Spine Imaging and Intervention,
Barrow Neurological Institute, Phoenix,
Arizona, USA

ANGELA GUARNIZO, MD
Assistant Professor, Radiology, Department of
Diagnostic Imaging, Hospital Universitario
Fundación Santa Fe de Bogota, Bogota,
Colombia

MAI-LAN HO, MD
Professor of Radiology, Vice Chair of
Operations and Innovation, Medical Director of
Radiology, Physician Director of Radiology
Informatics, Division Director of
Neuroradiology, University of Missouri,
Columbia, Missouri, USA

ANDREI I. HOLODNY, MD
Department of Radiology, Memorial Sloan
Kettering Cancer Center, New York, New York,
USA

MATTHEW T. HOUDEK, MD
Division of Orthopedic Oncology, Orthopedic
Surgery, Mayo Clinic, Rochester, Minnesota,
USA

JACK W. JENNINGS, MD, PhD
Mallinckrodt Institute of Radiology, Saint Louis,
Missouri, USA

KASSIE MCCULLAGH, MD
Assistant Professor, Division of
Neuroradiology, Department of Radiology,
The University of North Carolina, Chapel Hill,
North Carolina, USA

S. MOHAMMED KARIM, MD
Division of Orthopedic Oncology, Orthopedic
Surgery, Mayo Clinic, Rochester, Minnesota,
USA

SASAN KARIMI, MD
Department of Radiology, Memorial Sloan
Kettering Cancer Center, Department of
Radiology, Weill Cornell Medical College, New
York, New York, USA

MAJID A. KHAN, MD
Thomas Jefferson University Hospital,
Philadelphia, Pennsylvania, USA

ERIC LIS, MD
Department of Radiology, Weill Cornell
Medical College, New York, New York, USA

JONATHAN M. MORRIS, MD
Division of Neuroradiology, Department of
Radiology, Medical Director, Anatomic
Modeling Unit, Medical Director, Biomedical
and Scientific Visualization, Mayo Clinic,
Rochester, Minnesota, USA

KAMBIZ NAEL, MD
Professor, Division of Neuroradiology,
Department of Radiology, David Geffen School
of Medicine at UCLA, Los Angeles, California,
USA

LUIS NUNEZ, MD
Department of Diagnostic and Interventional
Imaging, The University of Texas Health
Science Center at Houston, McGovern Medical
School, Houston, Texas, USA

PUNEET S. PAWHA, MD
Associate Professor, Division of
Neuroradiology, Department of Radiology,
Icahn School of Medicine at Mount
Sinai Hospital, New York, New York,
USA

KYUNG K. PECK, PhD
Department of Radiology, Memorial Sloan
Kettering Cancer Center, New York, New York,
USA

PAULO PUAC-POLANCO, MD, MSc
Assistant Professor, Department of Radiology,
Radiation Oncology and Medical Physics,
University of Ottawa, Ottawa, Ontario, Canada

ROY RIASCOS, MD
Department of Diagnostic and Interventional
Imaging, The University of Texas Health
Science Center at Houston, McGovern Medical
School, Houston, Texas, USA

ANDRES RODRIGUEZ, MD
Department of Diagnostic and Interventional
Imaging, The University of Texas Health
Science Center at Houston, McGovern Medical
School, Houston, Texas, USA

FRANCISCO RIVAS RODRIGUEZ, MD
Clinical Associate Professor, Radiology,
Division of Neuroradiology, University of
Michigan, Michigan Medicine, C.S. Mott
Children's Hospital, Ann Arbor, Michigan, USA

PETER S. ROSE, MD
Division of Orthopedic Oncology, Orthopedic
Surgery, Mayo Clinic, Rochester, Minnesota,
USA

ATIN SAHA, MD, MS
Department of Radiology, Memorial Sloan
Kettering Cancer Center, Department of
Radiology, Weill Cornell Medical College,
New York, New York, USA

KAREN L. SALZMAN, MD
Professor, Department of Radiology, University
of Utah, Salt Lake City, Utah, USA

MICHAEL SCHECHT, MD
Assistant Professor, Division of
Neuroradiology, Department of Radiology,
Icahn School of Medicine at Mount
Sinai Hospital, New York, New York,
USA

LUBDHA M. SHAH, MD, MS
Professor, Department of Radiology, University of Utah, Salt Lake City, Utah, USA

DAVID TIMARAN-MONTENEGRO, MD, MSc
Department of Diagnostic and Interventional Imaging, The University of Texas Health Science Center at Houston, McGovern Medical School, Houston, Texas, USA

ANDERANIK TOMASIAN, MD
University of California Irvine, Orange, California, USA

CARLOS H. TORRES, MD, FRCPC, FCAR
Professor of Radiology, Department of Radiology, Radiation Oncology and Medical Physics, University of Ottawa, Ottawa, Ontario, Canada

ADAM WENTWORTH, MS
Department of Radiology, Anatomic Modeling Unit, Mayo Clinic, Rochester, Minnesota, USA

SEMA YILDIZ, MD
Assistant Professor, Division of Neuroradiology, Department of Radiology, Icahn School of Medicine at Mount Sinai Hospital, New York, New York, USA

CARLOS ZAMORA, MD, PhD
Associate Professor, Division of Neuroradiology, Department of Radiology, The University of North Carolina at Chapel Hill, Chapel Hill, North Carolina, USA

LUBDHA M. SHAH, MD, MS
Professor, Department of Radiology, University of Utah, Salt Lake City, Utah, USA

DAVID TIMARAN MONTENEGRO, MD, MSc
Department of Diagnostic and Interventional Imaging, The University of Texas Health Science Center at Houston, McGovern Medical School, Houston, Texas, USA

ANOERANIR TOMASIAN, MD
University of California Irvine, Orange, California, USA

CARLOS H. TORRES, MD, FRCPC, FCAR
Professor of Radiology, Department of Radiology, Radiation Oncology and Medical

Physics, University of Ottawa, Ontario, Canada

ADAM WENTWORTH, MS
Department of Radiology, Anatomic Modeling Unit, Mayo Clinic, Rochester, Minnesota, USA

SEMA YILDIZ, MD
Assistant Professor, Division of Neuroradiology, Department of Radiology, Icahn School of Medicine at Mount Sinai Hospital, New York, New York, USA

CARLOS ZAMORA, MD, PhD
Associate Professor, Division of Neuroradiology, Department of Radiology, The University of North Carolina at Chapel Hill, Chapel Hill, North Carolina, USA

Contents

The pediatric spine undergoes complex stages of development and growth, resulting in highly age-dependent physiology and variable susceptibility to certain pathologies. Optimal radiologic evaluation requires image acquisition tailored to the clinical history and an interpretive approach that accounts for demographic variations. In this article, the author discusses the diagnostic approach to pediatric spine masses, beginning with a discussion of normal anatomy and variants, clinical evaluation, and imaging techniques and protocols. The author then covers the major etiologies, imaging appearances, and mimics of pediatric spine masses in the following categories: congenital malformations, genetic syndromes, intramedullary, intradural, epidural, bone, and paraspinal lesions.

Spinal cord tumors are best identified by conventional MR imaging with contrast. Most intramedullary spinal cord tumors have characteristic MR imaging features that allow an accurate preoperative diagnosis. The spinal cord tumors reviewed in this article include the most common tumors, ependymomas and astrocytomas, as well as the less common tumors such as hemangioblastomas and metastases. Rare tumors such as primary CNS lymphoma and melanocytic tumors are also described. Advanced imaging techqniques of more common intramedullary tumors are also reviewed.

Most intradural tumors are located within the intradural extramedullary compartment, and the most common tumors are schwannomas and meningiomas. Other less common neoplasms include neurofibroma, solitary fibrous tumor, myxopapillary ependymoma, lymphoma, metastatic leptomeningeal disease, malignant peripheral nerve sheath tumor, and paraganglioma. Patients usually present with gait ataxia, radicular pain, and motor and sensory deficits due to chronic compressive myelopathy or radiculopathy. MRI is the modality of choice for detecting and evaluating intradural extramedullary spinal tumors. This imaging technique helps narrow the differential diagnosis and therefore decide treatment.

Radiologists play a primary role in identifying, characterizing, and classifying spinal metastases and can play a lifesaving role in the care of these patients by triaging those with instability to urgent spine surgery consultation. For this reason, an understanding of current treatment algorithms and principles of spinal stability in patients with cancer is vital for all who interpret spine studies. In addition, advances in imaging allow radiologists to provide more accurate diagnoses and characterize pathology, thereby improving patient safety.

Percutaneous image-guided minimally invasive thermal ablation and vertebral augmentation are robust techniques, part of the available armamentarium used by radiologists for the management of patients with spinal metastases. Such interventions have been established to be safe and effective in treatment of selected patients with vertebral metastases. Special attention to procedure techniques including choice of ablation modality, vertebral augmentation technique, and thermal protection is essential for improved patient outcomes.

Three-dimensional (3D) printing technology has proven to have many advantages in spine and sacrum surgery. 3D printing allows the manufacturing of life-size patient-specific anatomic and pathologic models to improve preoperative understanding of patient anatomy and pathology. Additionally, virtual surgical planning using medical computer-aided design software has enabled surgeons to create patient-specific surgical plans and simulate procedures in a virtual environment. This has resulted in reduced operative times, decreased complications, and improved patient outcomes. Combined with new surgical techniques, 3D-printed custom medical devices and instruments using titanium and biocompatible resins and polyamides have allowed innovative reconstructions.

Foreword
Spinal Tumors

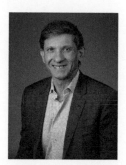

Suresh K. Mukherji, MD, MBA, FACR
Consulting Editor

I still remember when I first invited Dr Carlos H. Torres to guest edit this issue of *Neuroimaging Clinics* at a "prepandemic" meeting of the Radiological Society of North America. I was delighted when he accepted the invitation and suggested the topic of spinal tumors. Dr Torres is an internationally recognized neuroradiologist whom I would describe as a "Mover and Shaker" in global radiology. A summary of his accomplishments would require a separate issue of *Neuroimaging Clinics*, so suffice it to say we are privileged to have him as a Guest Editor,

This issue is singularly devoted to tumors involving the spine and spinal cord in both the adult and the pediatric population. There are articles covering advanced imaging techniques, such as DWI, DCE-MR imaging, and 3D printing, which emphasize technique and the specific impact of diagnosis, treatment, and management. There are

also articles devoted to percutaneous treatment and management of osseous metastases.

Finally, I would like to thank all the article authors for their outstanding contributions. These individuals are internationally recognized experts in their domain. The articles are state-of-the-art, and the image quality is superb. This is a unique issue of *Neuroimaging Clinics*, as there are very few concise books purely dedicated to spine tumors, and I thank Dr Torres for his vision, energy, and expertise in creating this outstanding issue.

Suresh K. Mukherji, MD, MBA, FACR
University of Illinois, ProScan Imaging
1185 West Carmel Drive, Suite D D1
Carmel, IN 46032, USA

E-mail address:
sureshmukherji@hotmail.com

Neuroimag Clin N Am 33 (2023) xv
https://doi.org/10.1016/j.nic.2023.05.003
1052-5149/23/© 2023 Published by Elsevier Inc.

Preface
Spinal Tumors

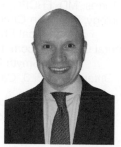

Carlos H. Torres, MD, FRCPC, FCAR
Editor

Cancer is the second most common cause of death in the United States, and the spine is the most common site of skeletal metastases, affecting approximately 40% of cancer patients, 20% of which become symptomatic. Cancer diagnosis used to have a poor prognosis; however, the advent of new therapies and treatment approaches has led to longer survival rates, even in patients with metastatic disease. Early diagnosis of a primary malignancy or metastatic disease is key to guide treatment and improve survival. To that effect, conventional and advanced imaging techniques, such as Diffusion-Weighted Imaging (DWI) and Dynamic Contrast-Enhanced (DCE) perfusion MR imaging, have become key tools not only for the identification and characterization of intradural and extradural spinal neoplasms but also for treatment planning and response.

Advances in MR techniques have improved the quality of spine DWI and Diffusion Tensor Imaging, leading to increased reproducibility and utilization. In addition, DWI has developed into a powerful adjunctive tool for the assessment of vertebral marrow lesions and intramedullary tumors. DCE-MR imaging, on the other hand, a well-established imaging technique for the assessment of brain neoplasms, is now being used for the diagnosis and treatment monitoring of patients with spinal metastases. DCE-MR imaging allows for early and accurate assessment of treatment failure versus viable tumor, information that is extremely important for the radiation oncologists and for the neurosurgeons.

Radiologists play a crucial role not only in identifying spinal metastases but also in triaging patients with spine instability to urgent consultation with spine surgery. Hence, an understanding of current treatment algorithms and principles of spinal stability in cancer patients is of utmost importance for all who interpret spine studies. For example, evidence-based management algorithms, such as NOMS, which incorporates four fundamental assessments: Neurologic, Oncologic, Mechanical instability, and Systemic disease, serve as frameworks to guide discussion and suggest best-available treatment options. Radiologists should also be familiar with and report the Spinal Instability Neoplastic Score and the Epidural Spinal Cord Compression grade to ensure clear communication with the treatment teams as well as timely patient care. In that regard, a multidisciplinary team, which includes radiologists, radiation oncologists, medical oncologists, and oncologic surgeons, is necessary when treating patients with cancer and spinal osseous metastatic disease. And although surgery and radiation therapy are considered the main treatment options, significant advances in percutaneous image-guided, minimally invasive oncologic interventions, such as thermal ablation and vertebral augmentation, allow radiologists to provide safe and timely patient care, while achieving pain palliation and local tumor control.

The first half of this issue is devoted to common and infrequent pediatric and adult intramedullary, intradural extramedullary, and extradural spinal tumors with an additional article on the tumor mimics that we need to recognize. This is followed by articles highlighting the role of advanced imaging techniques, such as DWI and DCE-MR imaging,

Neuroimag Clin N Am 33 (2023) xvii–xviii
https://doi.org/10.1016/j.nic.2023.05.002
1052-5149/23/© 2023 Published by Elsevier Inc.

in the assessment of spinal tumors, the current diagnosis and treatment of spine metastases, and the role of 3D printing technology in oncologic surgery of the spine and sacrum. I certainly hope you enjoy every article as much as I did while editing them and find this issue informative and helpful in clinical practice.

I would like to express my sincere gratitude to the extraordinary group of authors for their outstanding contributions and for their time and expertise. I would like to thank Karen Dino and John Vassallo at Elsevier for their assistance and flexibility in putting this issue together. Last,

but not least, I would like to thank Dr Suresh Mukherji for the opportunity to be the guest editor of this issue.

Carlos H. Torres, MD, FRCPC, FCAR
Department of Radiology, Radiation Oncology
and Medical Physics
Box 232, General Campus Room 1466e
501 Smyth Road
Ottawa, Ontario K1H 8L6, Canada

E-mail address:
catorres@toh.ca

Pediatric Spine Tumors and Dysontogenetic Masses

Mai-Lan Ho, MD

KEYWORDS

• Congenital • Development • Genetic • Mass • Pediatric • Spine • Tumor • Vascular

KEY POINTS

- The pediatric spine undergoes multiple stages of development and growth, resulting in highly age-dependent physiology and variable susceptibility to certain pathologies at each phase of life.
- Clinical symptoms are nonspecific and require correlation with a detailed evaluation of patient demographics, time course, neurologic deficits, and multisystem findings.
- In children, there is a higher incidence of congenital malformations and dysontogenetic masses related to developmental insults and/or genetic syndromes.
- Pediatric spine tumors can be evaluated using a space-based approach with differential diagnoses for intramedullary, intradural, epidural, bone, and paraspinal lesions.
- Tumor mimics to consider in the differential diagnosis include infection, inflammation, metabolic disease, infarction, and trauma.

INTRODUCTION

The pediatric spine undergoes multiple stages of development and growth from fetal life through infancy, childhood, and adolescence. This results in highly age-dependent physiology and unique susceptibility to certain pathologies at each phase of life. In children, there is a much higher incidence of congenital malformations and dysontogenetic masses, related to underlying developmental insults and/or genetic syndromes. Pathology of spinal tumors varies widely with demographic factors and includes benign, malignant, vascular, and dysplastic lesions. The radiologic differential also includes various tumor mimics such as infection, inflammation, metabolic disease, infarction, and trauma, which can present differently in children. Therefore, optimal radiologic evaluation of pediatric spine masses requires image acquisition tailored to the clinical history as well as an approach to interpretation that accounts for demographic variations. In this article, the author discusses the diagnostic approach to pediatric spine masses, beginning with a discussion of normal anatomy and variants, clinical evaluation, and imaging techniques and protocols. The author then covers the major etiologies, imaging appearances, and mimics of pediatric spine masses in the following categories: congenital malformations, genetic syndromes, intramedullary, intradural, epidural, bone, and paraspinal lesions. Although some developmental lesions and aggressive tumors demonstrate trans-spatial involvement, application of a compartmental approach helps greatly in evaluation of tumor origin, extent, and complications.

NORMAL ANATOMY AND VARIANTS

A basic understanding of spine development is helpful for classifying congenital anomalies and dysontogenetic masses. Major stages in fetal spine embryology include primary neurulation, secondary neurulation, segmentation, chondrification, primary ossification, and secondary ossification. Primary neurulation involves neural tube formation and disjunction of the neural ectoderm from the endothelial ectoderm. Secondary neurulation involves canalization and retrogressive differentiation of the caudal cell mass, which gives rise to the conus medullaris, filum terminale, and cauda equina nerve roots. Apoptosis of the distal neural

University of Missouri, University Hospital, 1 Hospital Drive, Columbia, MO 65212, USA
E-mail address: mailanho@gmail.com

Neuroimag Clin N Am 33 (2023) 375–388
https://doi.org/10.1016/j.nic.2023.04.002

tube during secondary neurulation enables differential growth of the vertebral column relative to the cord and nerve roots with relative ascent of the conus and dural sac. Developmental defects and/or masses in the distal spine can produce cord tension with restricted motion and growth, a phenomenon known as tethered cord syndrome.[1,2]

Spine segmentation involves the development of individual somites consisting of dermatomes, myotomes, and sclerotomes. The sclerotomes resegment and shift to yield a relative offset between the vertebral bodies and posterior elements. Vertebral ossification begins with chondrification and progresses through primary and secondary ossification stages, the latter involving closure of the epiphyses and apophyses with completion during adolescence. For radiology reporting, spine numbering should be performed with clear explanation of the numbering schema as well as reference to standard landmarks for surgical reference. Ideally, counting is performed from cranial to caudal, starting at the level of the cervical spine. In the setting of transitional anatomy, landmarks for assigning vertebral numbering include the orientation of transverse processes, ribs, iliolumbar ligaments, and lumbosacral plexus. Vertebral malformations can result from developmental variations in segmentation, ossification, and fusion.[3]

Marrow signal is an important feature to evaluate on magnetic resonance (MR) imaging and progresses through three major stages based on age. Stage I, from 0 to 1 month, shows biconvex vertebral bodies with central hypointensity in T1- and T2-weighted images, corresponding to the ossification centers, and prominent enhancement due to vascularity. The cartilaginous endplates are T1 hypointense and T2 hyperintense. Stage II, from 1 to 6 months, involves progressive T1 shortening of the vertebrae from peripheral to central with increasing T2 signal intensity. Stage III, after 7 months, involves T1 and T2 hyperintensity of the vertebral bodies with integration of the cartilaginous endplates, developing a squared appearance.[4]

CLINICAL EVALUATION

When evaluating a child with suspected spine pathology, patient age, gender, and race are important considerations that can impact the differential diagnosis. In the newborn, features suspicious for an underlying spine malformation include a high (within or above gluteal crease), deep, or asymmetric sacral dimple. Associated cutaneous changes such as hypertrichosis, discoloration (melanotic or vascular), open skin defect, dermal appendage, or mass are concerning for a spinal dysraphism. Low dimples (below the gluteal crease) and shallow dimples with intact overlying skin are common in infants and do not require further workup in the absence of neurologic symptoms. Distinction between open (not covered by skin) and closed (covered by skin) spinal dysraphisms are key to proper patient evaluation and management.[5]

For older children, the clinician should obtain a detailed clinical history with regard to onset (acute, subacute, chronic); course (monophasic, progressive); and symptoms (pain, weakness, numbness/tingling, bowel/bladder symptoms, restricted motion, spinal deformity). Unfortunately, the symptoms of pediatric spinal tumors are frequently nonspecific and can lead to delayed diagnosis with an emergent clinical presentation. Family history and exposures (recent illness, vaccinations, travel) are important to elicit and may suggest risk factors for disease. A complete physical examination should be performed to assess for a neurologic level as well as additional findings suggestive of a genetic or systemic condition. Findings can be supplemented by targeted laboratory testing such as cerebrospinal fluid (CSF) analysis, blood work, genetic testing, and/or biopsy.[6]

IMAGING TECHNIQUES AND PROTOCOLS

Conventional radiography has limited utility in evaluation of pediatric spine tumors but may be ordered as an initial screening examination to assess for acute trauma, bone remodeling, and osteoblastic or osteolytic lesions. Intraoperative fluoroscopy can be helpful for surgical guidance and localization. Following surgery, radiography is used for rapid assessment of hardware complications, spine alignment, and stability.[7]

Ultrasound (US) is a useful technique for fetal screening as well as neonatal spine imaging. Spine US in newborns is readily performed within the first 3 to 4 months of life, when the posterior elements have not yet fully ossified. If there is delayed ossification or a posterior osseous defect such as spina bifida, US may still be possible at 6 months or later. US enables evaluation of the dermis and sinus tracts, subcutaneous fat, epidural space, dura mater, spinal cord and nerve roots, and masses. US can also be helpful for interventional guidance, including lumbar punctures and spinal cord surgeries.[8]

Computed tomography (CT) provides the rapid assessment of osseous structures with high spatial resolution. Owing to the presence of ionizing radiation, CT is primarily used in the acute posttraumatic setting. With age-appropriate dose reduction, CT may also be used to evaluate bone detail for preoperative planning, intraoperative navigation, and anatomic coregistration with nuclear medicine (NM). Intravenous iodinated contrast should be administered if there is clinical suspicion for tumor or mass. However, given that CT is limited for evaluation of soft tissues and intradural structures, MR is typically preferred for initial imaging.[9]

MR imaging is used for detailed evaluation of fetal anomalies noted on US, including spine masses and malformations. After birth, MR is also the gold standard for pediatric spine imaging, providing exquisite bone marrow and soft tissue contrast. Given the length of the examination (20–60+ minutes depending on protocol), patient sedation and/or anesthesia may be required. For congenital malformations, a noncontrast protocol can be performed to include sagittal and axial T1- and T2-weighted sequences at a minimum. Fat-suppressed images can be added to confirm the presence of bulk fat in a lipomatous malformation or teratoma. Coronal T2 sequences are helpful for assessing complex segmentation anomalies, particularly in the setting of severe scoliosis. For detailed evaluation of tethered cord anatomy—including conus termination, nerve root morphology, and suspected sinus tracts—the authors recommend the use of a 3-dimensional balanced steady-state free precession sequence. Diffusion-weighted imaging (DWI) is useful for characterization of hypercellular tumor, inclusion cyst (dermoid/epidermoid), and inflammation/infection. Gradient-recalled echo (GRE) imaging can be used to assess areas of hemorrhage or mineralization. For suspected spine tumors or masses, intravenous gadolinium contrast is recommended. Macrocyclic agents are suggested to minimize the likelihood of gadolinium deposition with gadobutrol being the only Food and Drug Administration-approved agent for infants less than 2 years of age. For emergent cord compression, rapid sagittal sequences can be performed for initial screening and triage to the operating room.[10]

NM is useful for metabolic imaging, but has limited applications in pediatrics given the need for radiopharmaceutical administration. ^{18}F-fluorodeoxyglucose (^{18}F-FDG) positron emission tomography (PET) can be used for whole-body cancer staging to identify hypermetabolic tissues. Owing to the low spatial resolution and variable physiologic uptake in the spine, ^{18}F-FDG PET is most useful for assessment of large extraspinal tumors. For bone metastases, ^{18}F-sodium fluoride (^{18}F-NaF) PET or single-photon emission computed tomography using a blood pool agent such as technetium Tc [99m]-hydroxydiphosphonate can be helpful. Neuroendocrine tumor imaging can be performed with various radiolabeled somatostatin receptor analogs including octreotide, metaiodobenzylguanidine, fluorodopa, and dodecane tetraacetic acid (DOTA)-conjugated peptides. Several additional radiotracers are under research evaluation to assess different aspects of tumor biology but are not yet widely approved for pediatric clinical care.[11]

CONGENITAL MALFORMATIONS

Cystic lesions in the distal spine can result from vacuolization during secondary neurulation, affecting the conus (ventriculus terminalis) or filum terminale (filar cyst) (Fig. 1). These physiologic variants are generally asymptomatic and tend to involute with age. In the proximal spinal cord, a prominent central canal (≤ 2 mm) is a normal variant that should be distinguished from hydromyelia (>2 mm) and syringomyelia (eccentric and outside the central canal). Syrinx is a nonspecific term that can refer to any of the aforementioned entities and can be seen as a normal variant as well as secondary to disrupted CSF circulation in the setting of a spine malformation or tumor[12] (see Fig. 1).

Extramedullary CSF lesions may also arise developmentally. Spinal cord herniation can be associated with congenital dural deficiency. Arachnoid cysts or webs are most common in the dorsal spinal canal and can demonstrate thin delimiting walls with mild mass effect on the cord (Fig. 2). Neurenteric cysts are more common in the ventral spinal canal, associated with visceral abnormalities or sinus tracts[13] (see Fig. 2).

Lipomatous malformations consist of adipose tissue surrounding and often intimately associated with neural elements. It is common for fat to interdigitate along the placode and nerve roots, producing asymmetric displacement and rotation. An accurate description of this anatomy is critical to avoid inadvertent cord or nerve root injury during surgery. Simple lipomas are not associated with a spinal osseous defect and can be intradural extramedullary, intramedullary, or multifocal (Fig. 3). Lipomyeloschisis indicates a concurrent osteodural defect, possibly due to premature disjunction with mesenchyme directly contacting ependyma and stimulated to differentiate into adipose tissue. As a result, intradural fat blends smoothly into epidural and subcutaneous fat, without distinct boundaries. Dorsally, the spinal defect is covered by skin and subcutaneous fat. Therefore, classification relies on the location of the placode–lipoma interface relative to spinal canal: lipomyelocele (placode inside canal), lipomyelomeningocele (placode outside canal), or transitional (placode traversing osteodural defect)[14] (see Fig. 3).

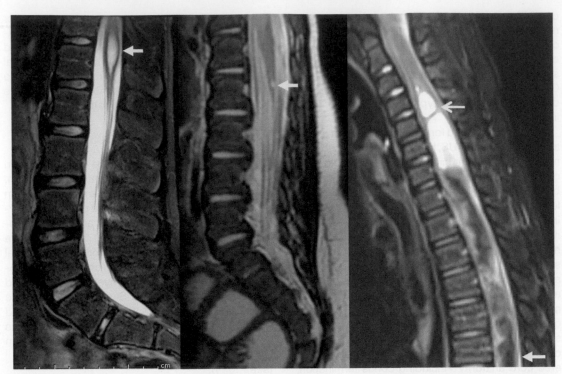

Fig. 1. Intramedullary cystic lesions. Sagittal T2-weighted MR shows ventriculus terminalis (*arrow*) in the conus medullaris (left panel), filar cyst (*arrow*) in the filum terminale (middle panel), and cord syrinx with septation (*thin arrow*) and turbulent bulk flow (*thick arrow*) (right panel).

Ectodermal inclusion cysts include epidermoid (squamous epithelium only) (Fig. 4A) and dermoid cysts (additional dermal appendages including hair, sebum, calcification). These can occur congenitally or following trauma or surgery with implantation of ectodermal elements (Fig. 4B). Teratomas are developmental tumors characterized by proliferation of all three germ cell layers with variable levels of differentiation and malignancy. Sacrococcygeal teratoma is the most common congenital spinal tumor, typically a mixed solid/cystic mass, with varying histologies including neuroglia, epithelium, cartilage, muscle, and bone. The Altman classification is defined by the fraction of extrapelvic versus intrapelvic involvement (types I–IV) with larger intrapelvic components portending a poorer prognosis due to lower clinical detection, greater likelihood of malignant transformation, and more difficult surgical resection[14] (Fig. 4C).

GENETIC SYNDROMES

Many spine tumors exhibit a familial predisposition that is suggestive of underlying genetic causality. This phenomenon is well demonstrated by the increased incidence of spinal abnormalities in tumor predisposition syndromes and neurocutaneous disorders. Depending on the molecular pathway

involved, there can be an increased risk of spine malformations, dysontogenetic masses, and benign or malignant tumors. As a result, patients with known genetic diagnoses require regular clinical and imaging surveillance.[15]

Neurofibromatosis type 1 is caused by mutations in the *NF1* tumor suppressor gene encoding neurofibromin. This acts as a tumor suppressor in cell cycle proliferation/differentiation and is expressed in various tissues including neurons, glia, vessels, connective tissue, and bone. Patients can have dysplastic, hamartomatous, or neoplastic lesions throughout the neuraxis. In the spine, common manifestations include multilevel dumbbell/plexiform neurofibromas as well as osteodural dysplasia with kyphoscoliosis, dural ectasia, and/or lateral meningoceles[16] (Fig. 5A).

Neurofibromatosis type 2 is caused by mutations in the *NF2* tumor suppressor gene encoding schwannomin, which supports cytoskeletal structure during neural development. In severe cases, patients can present with multiple schwannomas, meningiomas, ependymomas, and/or gliomas throughout the neuraxis[16] (Fig. 5B).

Von Hippel–Lindau disease results from mutations in the *VHL* tumor suppressor gene, which controls extracellular matrix formation and angiogenesis. Patients present with multisystem

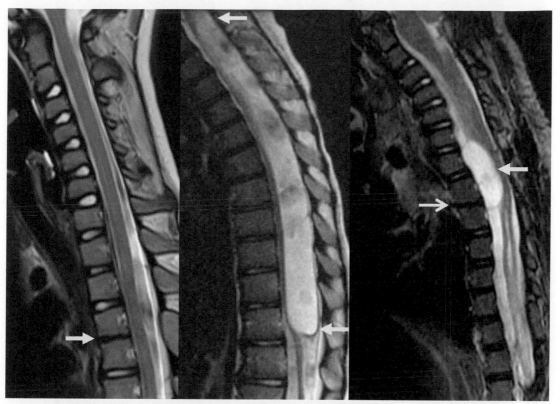

Fig. 2. Intradural cystic lesions. Sagittal T2-weighted MR shows cord herniation with anterior buckling abutting a hypoplastic disc (*arrow*) (left panel), arachnoid cyst with walled-off dorsal collection (*arrows*) compressing the cord (middle panel), and ventral neurenteric cyst (*thick arrow*) abutting vertebral and disc anomalies (*thin arrow*) with associated cord compression, distal myelomalacia and syrinx (right panel).

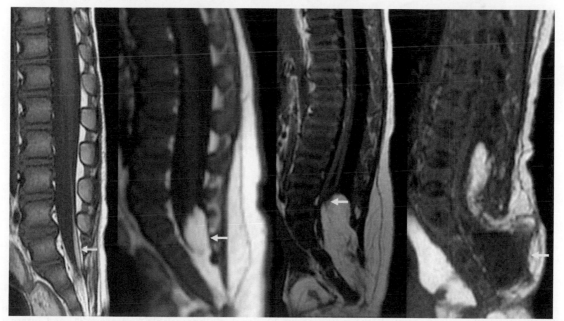

Fig. 3. Lipomatous malformations. Sagittal T1-weighted MR shows filum terminale fibrolipoma (*arrow*) with straightened morphology and slight elongation of conus medullaris (left panel), terminal lipoma (*arrow*) with no identifiable conus medullaris (second from left panel), lipomyelocele with placode–lipoma interface (*arrow*) within the spinal canal (third panel), and lipomyelomeningocele with placode–lipoma interface (*arrow*) outside the spinal canal (right panel).

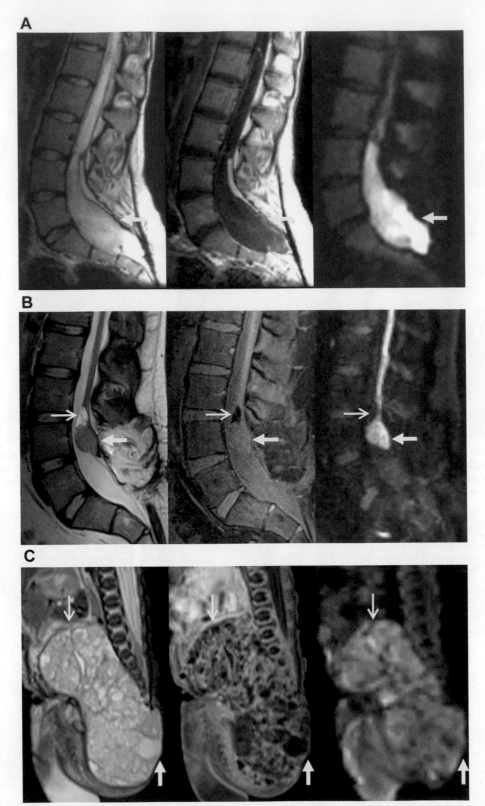

Fig. 4. Germinomatous lesions. Sagittal T2, post-contrast T1, and DWI MR show: (*A*) Expansile cystic lesion within the distal spinal canal demonstrating heterogeneous T2 signal, no appreciable enhancement, and internal restricted diffusion consistent with an epidermoid cyst (*arrows*). (*B*) Cord detethering surgery with postoperative dermoid containing bulk fat (*thin arrows*) and complex cyst with restricted diffusion (*thick arrows*). (*C*) Type II sacrococcygeal teratoma with heterogeneous solid and cystic tumor inside (*thin arrows*) and outside (*thick arrows*) the pelvis.

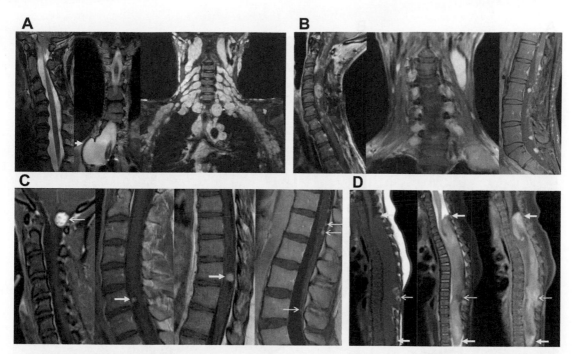

Fig. 5. Genetic syndromes. (A) Neurofibromatosis type 1. T2-weighted MR shows kyphoscoliosis (left panel), dural ectasia with right lateral meningocele (*arrow*) (central panel), and multilevel dumbbell and plexiform neurofibromas involving the bilateral foraminal/extraforaminal nerves, brachial plexi, and paraspinal nerves (right panel). (B) Neurofibromatosis type 2. Post-contrast T1-weighted MR shows multiple dural-based meningiomas and intramedullary ependymomas (left panel), as well as nerve root (central panel) and cauda equina schwannomas (right panel). (C) Von Hippel-Lindau. Post-contrast T1-weighted MR shows multifocal pial hemangioblastomas (*thin arrows*) with avid contrast enhancement, vascular engorgement, and tumoral cysts/cord edema associated with intramedullary lesions (*thick arrows*). (D) Spinal cord hamartoma with somatic *FGFR1* duplication. T1 (left panel), T2 with fat suppression (FS) (central panel), and post-contrast T1-weighted FS MR (right panel) show dorsal exophytic spinal cord mass (*thick arrows*) with heterogeneous signal and enhancement as well as focal osteodural defect (*thin arrows*).

angiomas, hamartomas, cysts, and tumors. Hemangioblastomas can be seen throughout the central nervous system, particularly in the cerebellum and spinal cord. These present as avidly enhancing lesions with prominent hypervascularity. Intramedullary lesions can demonstrate prominent cord edema and tumoral cysts[17] (Fig. 5C).

Spinal hamartomatous lesions can be associated with somatic cell cycle mutations as well as complex multisystem malformations. CLOVES is a recently described association: Congenital Lipomatous Overgrowth, Vascular malformations, Epidermal nevi, and Scoliosis/Skeletal/Spinal anomalies[18] (Fig. 5D).

INTRAMEDULLARY LESIONS

Primary cord tumors are classified according to histology and grade. Imaging features including cord asymmetry, heterogeneous signal, infiltrative margins, exophytic components, and skip/drop metastases can help to distinguish true tumors from mimics such as infection, inflammation, and ischemia. Long-standing tumors can also grow steadily with expansion and remodeling of the spinal canal.[19]

Spinal ependymomas arise from ependymal cells lining the central canal and are genetically distinct from intracranial ependymomas. They tend to be circumscribed and centrally located within the spinal cord. These are hypervascular tumors with avid enhancement and variable cystic/hemorrhagic degeneration, yielding tumoral edema, cysts, and siderosis.[20]

Astrocytomas originate from astrocytic glial cells, appearing more infiltrative and eccentric. Histologic subtypes include pilocytic, fibrillary, pilomyxoid, pleomorphic, anaplastic, and glioblastoma. Lower grade tumors grow slowly with fusiform long-segment cord expansion, T2-hyperintense signal, and variable enhancement (Fig. 6A). Higher grade tumors demonstrate greater neovascularity, irregular margins, and heterogeneous signal with necrosis and hemorrhage[20] (Fig. 6B).

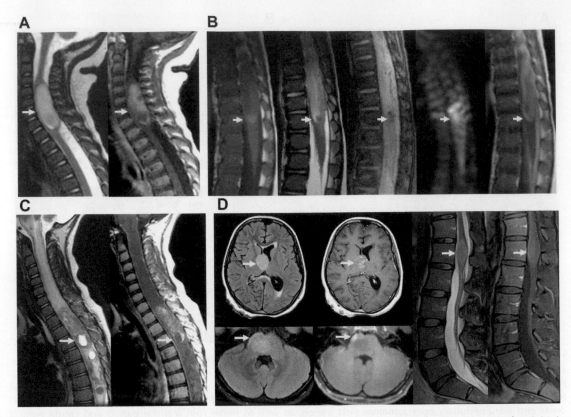

Fig. 6. Intramedullary tumors. (A) Astrocytoma. Sagittal T2 (left panel) and post-contrast T1-weighted (right panel) MR show eccentric fusiform cord mass with heterogeneous signal and enhancement (*arrows*). (B) Glioblastoma. Sagittal T1, T2, gradient-recalled echo (GRE), DWI, and post-contrast T1-weighted MR (left to right panels) show an expansile distal cord tumor with heterogeneous enhancement, hypervascularity, internal necrosis/hemorrhage, restricted diffusion, and leptomeningeal dissemination (*arrows*). (C) Ganglioglioma. Sagittal T2 (left panel) and post-contrast T1-weighted (right panel) MR show long-segment expansile cord lesion with heterogeneous enhancement, cysts, and hemorrhage (*arrows*). (D) Diffuse midline glioma. Axial fluid-attenuated inversion recovery (FLAIR) and post-contrast T1-weighted MR of the brain (left panel) show expansile heterogeneously enhancing lesions of the right thalamus and pons (*arrows*). Sagittal T2 and post-contrast T1-weighted FS MR of the lumbar spine (right panel) show expansile infiltrative and heterogeneously enhancing mass in the conus (*arrows*).

Gangliogliomas are mixed tumors composed of both astrocytes and neural cells. Small tumors are usually homogeneous and slow growing with minimal edema and enhancement. Larger lesions can appear heterogeneous with mild edema, patchy peripheral/internal enhancement, tumoral cysts, and calcifications[20] (Fig. 6C).

Diffuse midline gliomas are World Health Organization (WHO) grade 4 tumors molecularly characterized by histone *H3 K27M* alterations, often in association with tumor predisposition syndromes (constitutional mismatch repair deficiency syndrome, Lynch, Li-Fraumeni). These are aggressive midline tumors affecting children and young adults. On imaging, there is often multifocal tumor infiltration, necrosis, and hemorrhage. Lesions can involve the deep gray structures, brainstem, cerebellum, and spinal cord[21] (Fig. 6D).

INTRADURAL LESIONS

Intradural tumors can grow progressively with smooth bony expansion and remodeling of the spinal canal and neural foramina. Myxopapillary ependymoma is a WHO grade 2 subtype of ependymoma that arises from the distal neural elements (conus medullaris, filum terminale, cauda equina). Tumors classically appear lobular or sausage-like with a circumscribed and elongated morphology, avid contrast enhancement, hypervascularity, and cystic/hemorrhagic transformation[22] (Fig. 7A).

Diffuse leptomeningeal glioneuronal tumor is a low-grade oligodendroglial-like tumor that presents throughout the leptomeningeal space without obvious primary lesion. On imaging, multifocal cystic lesions are present throughout the subarachnoid space with variable leptomeningeal thickening/nodularity, enhancement, and bone remodeling. Occasionally, intra-axial lesions may be observed in the spinal cord[21] (Fig. 7B).

Drop metastases in the spine can be seen with leptomeningeal carcinomatosis from various primary pathologies including medulloblastoma, ependymoma, rhabdoid tumors, choroid plexus tumors, and germ cell tumors. These can present as multinodular or thick confluent deposits over the pial cord surface and cauda equina nerve roots.[23] (Fig. 7C)

Peripheral nerve sheath tumors present as nodular or fusiform lesions oriented along the exiting nerve roots or cauda equina. Lesions that occur in isolation usually represent schwannomas. For

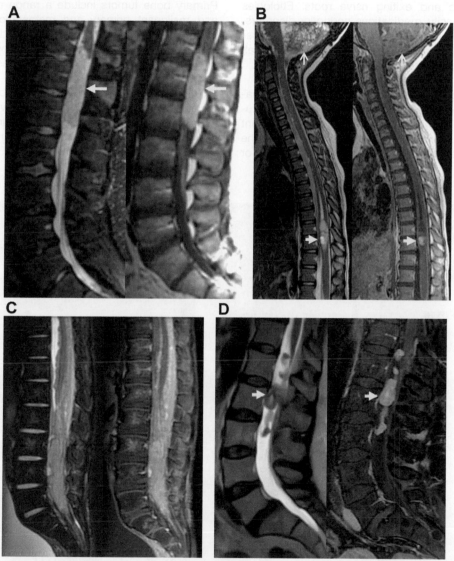

Fig. 7. Intradural tumors. (A) Myxopapillary ependymoma. Sagittal T2 FS (left panel) and post-contrast T1-weighted MR (right panel) show ovoid enhancing intradural lesion (arrows) encasing the proximal filum terminale and cauda equina nerve roots, producing mild deformation of the conus. (B) Diffuse leptomeningeal glioneuronal tumor. Sagittal T2 (left panel) and post-contrast T1-weighted (right panel) MR show diffuse cystic and nodular enhancing lesions throughout the subarachnoid space (thin arrows) with single intra-axial mass in the midthoracic cord (thick arrows). (C) Drop metastases from medulloblastoma. Sagittal T2 FS (left panel) and post-contrast T1-weighted FS (right panel) MR of the thoracic and lumbar spine show diffuse nodular and confluent enhancing tissue coating the spinal cord and cauda equina nerve roots. (D) Schwannomatosis. Sagittal T2 (left panel) and post-contrast T1-weighted FS (right panel) MR show plexiform schwannomas involving multiple cauda equina nerve roots (arrows).

atypical or multiple lesions, consider genetic testing for both germline and somatic variants[24] (**Fig. 7**D).

EPIDURAL LESIONS

Epidural lipomatosis refers to increased fat deposition within the epidural space. On imaging, the finding is often diffuse but most severe in the lumbar spine with potential compression of the distal thecal sac and exiting nerve roots. Etiologies include obesity, medications, endocrine disorders, and idiopathic. Multifocal involvement may be present with increased subcutaneous, mediastinal, visceral, mesenteric, and retroperitoneal fat.[25] (**Fig. 8**A)

On imaging, infectious phlegmon or inflammatory pseudomasses can occasionally mimic tumors.[26] (**Fig. 8**B-C) Various benign and malignant primary tumors and metastases can involve the epidural space, typically originating in bone or paraspinal tissues with subsequent epidural invasion. These lesions can present as oncologic emergencies with cord compression in the setting of minimal trauma, slight growth, or transient edema following radiation therapy[27] (**Fig. 8**D).

BONE LESIONS

Primary bone tumors include a range of benign and malignant primary and metastatic lesions. Depending on age and history, the differential diagnosis can include infection (discitis, osteomyelitis), inflammation (spondyloarthropathies, chronic recurrent multifocal osteomyelitis), and ischemia (bone infarcts, avascular necrosis). For bone neoplasms and their mimics, associated volumetric expansion of the vertebrae and epidural space can predispose to cord compression and neurologic deterioration.[28]

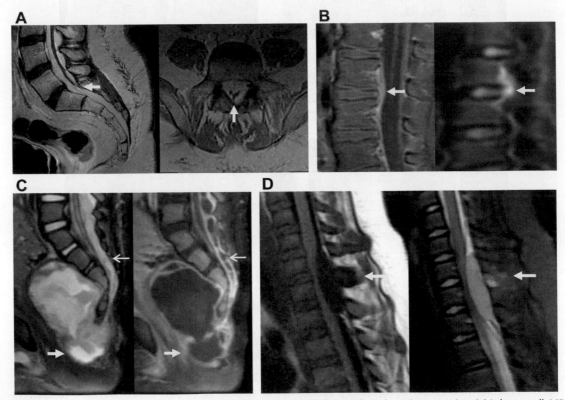

Fig. 8. Epidural lesions. (*A*) Epidural lipomatosis. Sagittal T1 (left panel) and axial T1-weighted (right panel) MR show diffusely increased epidural and subcutaneous fat with compression of the distal thecal sac (*arrows*). (*B*) Salmonella osteomyelitis. Sagittal post-contrast T1 FS (left panel) and DWI MR (right panel) show posterior disc and ventral epidural enhancement with restricted diffusion (*arrows*). (*C*) Sacrococcygeal teratoma complicated by epidural abscess. Sagittal T2 FS (left panel) and post-contrast T1-weighted FS MR (right panel) show heterogeneous presacral mass (*thick arrows*) with multilevel neural foraminal and epidural extension (*thin arrows*). (*D*) Ewing sarcoma presenting with hemorrhage after trauma. Sagittal T1 (left panel) and sagittal T2-weighted FS MR (right panel) show heterogeneous tumor infiltration of the C7 spinous process (*arrows*) with extension into the dorsal epidural space causing cord compression.

Osteochondroma is a benign osteocartilaginous exostosis that can be sessile or pedunculated. The cortex and marrow are continuous with parent bone. Multiple osteochondromas can be seen in the setting of hereditary multiple exostoses[29] (Fig. 9A).

Osteoid osteoma and osteoblastoma are benign osteoid-producing tumors that usually present in the posterior elements of the spine, distinguished by relative size (less or greater than 1.5 cm, respectively). The central nidus is usually lucent but may show variable amounts of sclerosis. There is a prominent surrounding zone of reactive edema, inflammation, and ossification in the bone and soft tissues. This flare phenomenon can mimic infection,

trauma, or malignancy. Imaging plays a crucial role in identification of the underlying nidus[29] (Fig. 9B).

Langerhans cell histiocytosis represents a clonal proliferation of histiocytes with formation of eosinophilic granulomatous skeletal lesions. Spinal involvement is more common in children and often presents with lytic bone destruction, pathologic vertebral fractures with near-complete loss of height (vertebra plana), and extraosseous extension. Additional lesions can be seen throughout the skeleton, hypothalamic-pituitary axis, skin, and viscera[29] (Fig. 9C).

Aneurysmal bone cyst is a bone tumor characterized by multiple expansile cysts containing blood–fluid levels, separated by well-defined

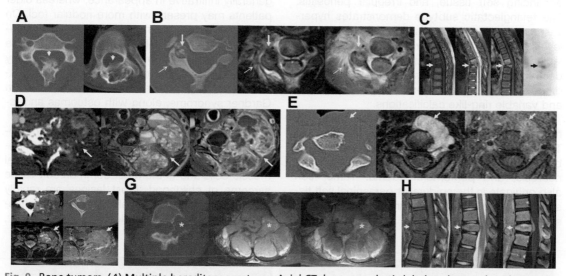

Fig. 9. Bone tumors. (A) Multiple hereditary exostoses. Axial CT shows exophytic lobulated osteochondromas (arrows) arising from the cervical and thoracic posterior elements with corticomedullary continuity and severe cord compression. (B) Osteoid osteoma. Axial CT (left panel), T2 FS (central panel) and post-contrast T1-weighted FS MR (right panel) show mixed lytic/sclerotic nidus in the right cervical facet joint (thick arrows) with surrounding reactive bone and soft tissue inflammation (thin arrows). (C) Langerhans cell histiocytosis. Sagittal T1 (left panel), T2 FS (second panel), post-contrast T1-weighted FS (third panel) MR, and positron emission tomography (right panel) show marrow signal changes and pathologic compression fractures in the midthoracic spine with vertebra plana (arrows), kyphosis, retropulsion, and epidural extension. (D) Aneurysmal bone cyst. Axial CT with contrast (left panel), T2 (central panel) and post-contrast T1-weighted FS MR (right panel) show a multilocular left paraspinal mass (arrows) with peripheral/septal enhancement, multiple fluid-blood levels, and extension to the lateral epidural space. (E) Chordoma. Axial CT (left panel), T2 FS (central panel), and post-contrast T1-weighted FS MR (right panel) show left paramedian cervical spine mass (arrows) with lobulated exophytic morphology, bone destruction, T2-hyperintense signal, patchy enhancement, and neural foraminal/epidural extension. (F) Telangi ectatic osteosarcoma. Axial CT with contrast in soft tissue and bone windows (top row) show infiltrative exophytic mass (arrows) arising from the left cervical spine with hypervascular solid enhancement, necrosis, and coarse calcifications. Axial T2 and post-contrast T1-weighted FS MR (bottom row) show bone destruction and neural foraminal/epidural extension. (G) Ewing sarcoma. Axial CT (left panel), T2 FS (central panel), and post-contrast T1-weighted FS MR (right panel) show infiltrative lumbar spine mass with irregular central lysis (asterisks), posterior sclerosis and periostitis, and multifocal osseous breakthrough. Tumor shows heterogeneous enhancement, necrosis, and inflammation with circumferential epidural and neural foraminal involvement, severe cord compression, and involvement of bilateral paraspinal and left psoas muscles. (H) Lymphoma. Sagittal T1 (left panel), T2 FS (central panel), and post-contrast T1-weighted FS MR (right panel) show lymphomatous infiltration of three midthoracic vertebrae with pathologic compression fracture (arrows), focal kyphosis, epidural tumor extension, and cord compression.

bone septations and variable solid components. Lesions can be primary or secondary to another tumor, such as giant cell tumor or osteoblastoma[30] (Fig. 9D).

Chordoma is a malignant tumor arising from notochordal remnants in the paramedian spine, which can involve multiple vertebrae and intervening discs. On CT, tumors show lytic osseous destruction and dystrophic calcifications. Prominent soft tissue components demonstrate variable signal, enhancement, necrosis, and diffusion restriction, based on tumor differentiation[30] (Fig. 9E).

Sarcomas are malignant connective tissue tumors that vary in appearance based on the underlying histology. Osteosarcoma is composed of osteoid matrix with dense sclerosis, avidly enhancing soft tissue, and irregular periostitis. The telangiectatic subtype demonstrates hypervascular angiomatous tissue with fluid–blood levels (Fig. 9F). Chondrosarcoma consists of cartilaginous matrix with lobulated margins, lytic bone destruction, T2-hyperintense MR signal, facilitated diffusion, avid enhancement, internal septations, and variable ring-like calcifications.[30]

Ewing sarcoma family tumors are primitive neuroectodermal tumors with aggressive morphology. These often involve the spine with permeative bone destruction, mixed lysis/sclerosis, internal necrosis, and peritumoral edema. Tumor can also originate in the epidural or paraspinal soft tissues and demonstrate perineural patterns of spread[30] (Fig. 9G).

Lymphoproliferative disorders, including lymphoma and leukemia, can yield primary bone lesions as well as secondary bone metastases or systemic disease. Bone involvement is frequently permeative with marrow infiltration, irregular cortical breakthrough, perivertebral soft tissue, and pathologic fractures[30] (Fig. 9H).

PARASPINAL LESIONS

Lesions that can involve the paraspinal space include soft tissue tumors, neurogenic tumors, and bone tumors with extraosseous extension. Desmoid fibromatosis is a benign but locally aggressive tumor with a high rate of recurrence following surgical excision. Pediatric lesions are generally infiltrative in appearance, whereas older patients may present with more nodular foci. On MR, fibromas are prominently T1 and T2 hypointense with low-level delayed enhancement. These characteristics can overlap with inflammatory fibrous lesions and benign or malignant fibrous tumors. Multifocal plaque-like fibromas are seen in Gardner syndrome, along with osteomas and familial adenomatous polyposis[31] (Fig. 10A).

Soft tissue sarcomas vary widely in imaging appearances according to histology and grade. Rhabdomyosarcoma arises from primitive skeletal muscle cells and is the most common soft tissue sarcoma of childhood. Most lesions are rapidly growing and invasive with heterogeneous enhancement, restricted diffusion reflecting hypercellularity,

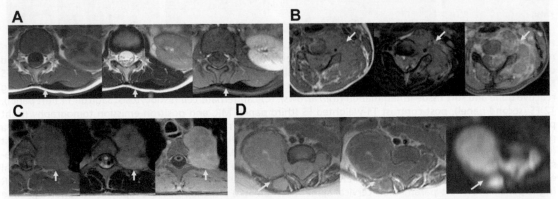

Fig. 10. Paraspinal tumors. (*A*) Desmoid fibromatosis. Axial T1 (left panel), T2 (central panel), and post-contrast T1-weighted FS MR (right panel) show a plaque-like lesion (*arrows*) in the left lumbar paraspinal musculoaponeurosis with diffusely hypointense signal and minimal enhancement. (*B*) Rhabdomyosarcoma. Axial T1 (left panel), T2 FS (central panel), and post-contrast T1-weighted FS MR (right panel) show a multilobulated left cervical paraspinal mass (*arrows*) with heterogeneous enhancement, bone infiltration, vertebral artery encasement, neural foraminal/epidural extension, and cord compression. (*C*) Paraganglioma. Axial T1 (left panel), T2 FS (central panel), and post-contrast T1-weighted FS MR (right panel) show lobulated left thoracic paraspinal mass (*arrows*) with avid enhancement, internal flow voids, and smooth bone erosions. (*D*) Neuroblastoma. Axial T2 (left panel), post-contrast T1-weighted MR (central panel) and metaiodobenzylguanidine (MIBG) single-photon emission computed tomography (right panel) show a lobulated heterogeneous and hypermetabolic mass in the right lumbar paraspinal region (*arrows*), extending through the right neural foramen through spinal canal and left neural foramen, and causing severe cord compression.

and areas of necrosis (Fig. 10B). Leiomyosarcoma shows smooth muscle differentiation derived from blood vessels, soft tissue, or skin with hypervascularity and variable intratumoral hemorrhage. Synovial sarcomas occur in close proximity to joints with admixed hemorrhage, necrosis, and calcification.[32]

Paraspinal peripheral nerve sheath tumors can occur sporadically or in association with a genetic syndrome. Interconnected lesions can be seen in the setting of neurofibromatosis type 1 (plexiform neurofibromas) or schwannomatosis (plexiform schwannomas).[33]

Paragangliomas arise from paraganglion cells in sympathetic or parasympathetic chains. They demonstrate enhancement and hypervascularity, along with cystic components and calcification in larger lesions. Large paraspinal tumors can progressively erode and remodel bone. Multiple paragangliomas can occur synchronously or metachronously in multiple paraganglioma syndromes, multiple endocrine neoplasia, neurofibromatosis type 1, and von Hippel-Lindau[33] (Fig. 10C).

Neuroblastic tumors arise from primitive neural crest cells located in the posterior mediastinum and retroperitoneum. The classification from benign to malignant includes ganglioneuroma, ganglioneuroblastoma, and neuroblastoma. Neuroblastoma is the most common extracranial solid malignancy in children. Small lesions can appear localized and defined, whereas larger lesions are aggressively infiltrative with hemorrhage, necrosis, and calcification. Paraspinal lesions can extend perineurally into the epidural space and infiltrate or metastasize to bone (Fig. 10D).

SUMMARY

The pediatric spine undergoes multiple stages of development and growth, resulting in highly age-dependent physiology and variable susceptibility to certain pathologies at each phase of life. Clinical symptoms are nonspecific and require correlation with a detailed evaluation of patient demographics, time course, neurologic deficits, and multisystem findings. In children, there is a higher incidence of congenital malformations and dysontogenetic masses related to developmental insults and/or genetic syndromes. Pediatric spine tumors can be evaluated using a space-based approach with differential diagnoses for intramedullary, intradural, epidural, bone, and paraspinal lesions. Although some developmental lesions and aggressive tumors demonstrate trans-spatial involvement, utilization of a compartmental approach helps greatly in evaluation of tumor origin, extent, and complications. Tumor mimics to consider in the differential diagnosis include infection, inflammation, metabolic disease, infarction, and trauma.

CLINICS CARE POINTS

- Pediatric spine anatomy and physiology are dynamic and age-dependent.
- In children, there is a higher incidence of congenital malformations and genetic syndromes.
- Clinical symptoms can be nonspecific and lead to delayed diagnosis.
- A space-based imaging approach is helpful in evaluating pediatric spine tumors and mimics.

DISCLOSURES

The author has nothing to disclose.

REFERENCES

1. Copp AJ, Stanier P, Greene ND. Neural tube defects: recent advances, unsolved questions, and controversies. Lancet Neurol 2013;12(8):799–810.
2. Nabizadeh N, Dimar JR. Congenital spine deformities: timing of insult during development of the spine in utero. Spine Deform 2022;10(1):31–44.
3. Thawait GK, Chhabra A, Carrino JA. Spine segmentation and enumeration and normal variants. Radiol Clin North Am 2012;50(4):587–98.
4. Chan BY, Gill KG, Rebsamen SL, et al. MR Imaging of Pediatric Bone Marrow. Radiographics 2016; 36(6):1911–30.
5. Wilson P, Hayes E, Barber A, et al. Screening for Spinal Dysraphisms in Newborns With Sacral Dimples. Clin Pediatr (Phila). 2016;55(11):1064–70.
6. Wilne S, Walker D. Spine and spinal cord tumours in children: a diagnostic and therapeutic challenge to healthcare systems. Arch Dis Child Educ Pract Ed 2010;95(2):47–54.
7. Goodwin ML, Buchowski JM, Sciubba DM. Why X-rays? The importance of radiographs in spine surgery. Spine J 2022;22(11):1759–67.
8. Alvarado E, Leach J, Caré M, et al. Pediatric Spinal Ultrasound: Neonatal and Intraoperative Applications. Semin Ultrasound CT MR 2017;38(2):126–42.
9. Larson AN, Schueler BA, Dubousset J. Radiation in Spine Deformity: State-of-the-Art Reviews. Spine Deform 2019;7(3):386–94.
10. Sorantin E, Robl T, Lindbichler F, et al. MRI of the neonatal and paediatric spine and spinal canal. Eur J Radiol 2008;68(2):227–34.
11. Biassoni L, Easty M. Paediatric nuclear medicine imaging. Br Med Bull 2017;123(1):127–48.

12. Naidich TP, Schefflein J, Cedillo MA, et al. The Distal Spine: Normal Embryogenesis and Derangements Leading to Malformation. Neuroimaging Clin N Am 2019;29(3):385–409.

13. Grimme JD, Castillo M. Congenital anomalies of the spine. Neuroimaging Clin N Am 2007;17(1):1–16.

14. Rossi A, Biancheri R, Cama A, et al. Imaging in spine and spinal cord malformations. Eur J Radiol 2004;50(2):177–200.

15. Sood S, Hryhorczuk AL, Rissmiller J, et al. Spectrum of Syndromic Disorders Associated with Pediatric Tumors: Evolving Role of Practical Imaging Assessment. Radiol Clin North Am 2017;55(4):869–93.

16. Tamura R. Current Understanding of Neurofibromatosis Type 1, 2, and Schwannomatosis. Int J Mol Sci 2021;22(11):5850.

17. Aronow ME, Wiley HE, Gaudric A, et al. VON HIPPEL-LINDAU DISEASE: Update on Pathogenesis and Systemic Aspects. Retina 2019;39(12):2243–53.

18. Garzon MC, Huang JT, Enjolras O, et al. Vascular malformations. Part II: associated syndromes. J Am Acad Dermatol 2007;56(4):541–64.

19. Kandemirli SG, Reddy A, Hitchon P, et al. Intramedullary tumours and tumour mimics. Clin Radiol 2020;75(11):876.e17–32.

20. Auguste KI, Gupta N. Pediatric intramedullary spinal cord tumors. Neurosurg Clin N Am 2006;17(1):51–61.

21. Louis DN, Perry A, Wesseling P, et al. The 2021 WHO Classification of Tumors of the Central Nervous System: a summary. Neuro Oncol 2021;23(8):1231–51.

22. Kresbach C, Neyazi S, Schüller U. Updates in the classification of ependymal neoplasms: The 2021 WHO Classification and beyond. Brain Pathol 2022;32(4):e13068.

23. Marrazzo A, Cacchione A, Rossi S, et al. Intradural Pediatric Spinal Tumors: An Overview from Imaging to Novel Molecular Findings. Diagnostics 2021;11(9):1710.

24. Karsy M, Guan J, Sivakumar W, et al. The genetic basis of intradural spinal tumors and its impact on clinical treatment. Neurosurg Focus 2015;39(2):E3.

25. Kim K, Mendelis J, Cho W. Spinal Epidural Lipomatosis: A Review of Pathogenesis, Characteristics, Clinical Presentation, and Management. Global Spine J 2019;9(6):658–65.

26. Rossi A. Pediatric spinal infection and inflammation. Neuroimaging Clin N Am 2015;25(2):173–91.

27. Kumar R, Giri PJ. Pediatric extradural spinal tumors. Pediatr Neurosurg 2008;44(3):181–9.

28. Sciubba DM, Hsieh P, McLoughlin GS, et al. Pediatric tumors involving the spinal column. Neurosurg Clin N Am 2008;19(1):81–92.

29. Shah J, Gandhi D, Chauhan A, et al. Imaging Review of Pediatric Benign Osteocytic Tumors and Latest Updates on Management. J Clin Med 2021;10(13):2823.

30. Kim HJ, McLawhorn AS, Goldstein MJ, et al. Malignant osseous tumors of the pediatric spine. J Am Acad Orthop Surg 2012;20(10):646–56.

31. Mills MK, Shah LM. Imaging of the perivertebral space. Radiol Clin North Am 2015;53(1):163–80.

32. Davis WL, Harnsberger HR. CT and MRI of the normal and diseased perivertebral space. Neuroradiology 1995;37(5):388–94.

33. Carter BW, Lichtenberger JP 3rd. Imaging of the Posterior/Paravertebral Mediastinum. Radiol Clin North Am 2021;59(2):243–9.

Conventional and Advanced Imaging of Spinal Cord Tumors

Lubdha M. Shah, MD, MS*, Karen L. Salzman, MD

KEYWORDS

- Spinal cord tumor • Intramedullary tumor • Magnetic resonance imaging • Diffusion • Perfusion

KEY POINTS

- Gliomas including ependymomas and astrocytomas are the most common intramedullary spinal cord tumors accounting for 80% of primary spinal cord tumors.
- Ependymomas are typically well-defined, concentric, expansile T2 hyperintense lesions with intense enhancement.
- Astrocytomas are typically diffusely infiltrative expansile masses eccentric to the central spinal canal with variable enhancement patterns.
- Less common primary spinal cord tumors such as hemangioblastoma are often associated with extensive edema and prominent vessels.
- Although technically challenging, advanced imaging techniques have a great potential for future directions.

CONVENTIONAL IMAGING OF SPINAL CORD TUMORS

Intramedullary tumors account for 20% to 30% of all primary intradural tumors; however, spinal cord tumors are uncommon, accounting for approximately 2% to 4% of all primary central nervous system tumors.[1,2] Primary intra-axial tumors are usually derived from neuroepithelial tissue, typically glial cells. Depending on the cell of origin, spinal cord tumors originate from different components of the spinal cord. Astrocytic tumors tend to originate from the peripheral white matter, whereas tumors of neuronal origin tend to originate from the central gray matter. Gliomas, such as astrocytoma and ependymoma, account for 80% of all intramedullary tumors, whereas hemangioblastomas and metastases comprise 3% to 8% and 2%, respectively.[2,3] Other rare tumors include primary central nervous system (CNS) lymphomas and melanocytic tumors.

MR imaging is the modality of choice to evaluate intramedullary lesions due to the superb soft tissue contrast and spatial resolution. In addition to the different features on T1-weighted and T2-weighted sequences in sagittal and axial planes, contrast-enhanced sequences can improve delineation of the extent of a mass and provide guidance for surgical biopsy, resection, or stereotactic radiosurgery.[4] Assessment of the entire neuroaxis may be useful to evaluate for skip lesions or drop metastases, which affect treatment decisions including biopsy targets and therapeutic goals.

EPENDYMOMA

Ependymoma is the most common intramedullary tumor in adults and accounts for 60% to 70% of all intramedullary glial tumors.[2] In the pediatric population, ependymomas are more common in the setting of neurofibromatosis type 2.[5,6] Spinal ependymomas have a 1:2 female:male ratio and present during the third to sixth decades.[7] Ependymomas are classified according to a combination of histopathological and molecular features as well as anatomic site, thus dividing them into molecular

Department of Radiology, University of Utah, 30 North 1900 East, Room#1A71, Salt Lake City, UT, USA
* Corresponding author.
E-mail address: lubdha.shah@hsc.utah.edu

Neuroimag Clin N Am 33 (2023) 389-406
https://doi.org/10.1016/j.nic.2023.03.001
1052-5149/23/© 2023 Elsevier Inc. All rights reserved.

groups across the supratentorial, posterior fossa, and spinal compartments. Classic spinal ependymomas, myxopapillary ependymomas, and subependymomas form different methylation groups.[8] An aggressive spinal ependymoma characterized by early neuroaxial dissemination, an anaplastic morphology, and MYCN gene amplification has been reported.[9,10]

Ependymomas are central in location because they originate from ependymal cells lining the central canal and, most commonly, in the cervical (45% of cases)[7] and thoracic segments.[11] Displacement rather than infiltration of the adjacent neural tissue by these lesions facilitates surgical resection[12] (Fig. 1). These well-defined, concentric, expansile intramedullary lesions are isointense to hypointense on T1-weighted imaging (T1WI) and hyperintense on T2-weighted imaging (T2WI). They typically exhibit well-defined intense enhancement, with homogeneous (75%), heterogeneous, rim, or nodular pattern.[13,14] The enhancing portion is associated with extensive edema. Tumor-associated cysts are common, reported in 88% in a case series of 59 patients.[13] The cysts may be intratumoral (22%–52.2%) and/or polar (21.7%–90%).[12,15,16] Altered cerebrospinal fluid (CSF) flow can result in syringomyelia, which is often seen (10%–50%).[14] As ependymomas can bleed, there may be T1 hyperintense foci. A T2 hypointense rim at the superior and/or inferior margins (cap sign) due to hemosiderin[13] has been reported in 20% to 45% of cases[12] (Fig. 2).

Myxopapillary ependymoma is an intradural, extramedullary mass, originating from ependymal cells in the filum terminale. It is the most common primary neoplasm of the conus medullaris and cauda equina, largely affecting young and middle-aged adults with a mean age of 36 years.[12] The World Health Organization (WHO) recently changed it from grade 1 to grade 2 because its likelihood of recurrence is similar to conventional spinal ependymoma.[9] The scattered pools of clear mucin on histopathology and the shiny surface at gross pathology correlate with high signal intensity on T2WI (Fig. 3). The "papillary" portion of the name corresponds to the papillary arrangement of tumor cells around a vascular core.[12,17]

Subependymoma is a WHO grade 1 tumor, accounting for 1% to 2% of adult spinal ependymal tumors. Subependymomas are identified with methylome studies but the molecular classification does not provide added clinicopathological utility.[8] Spinal subependymomas are expansile, lobulated T1 hypointense/isointense, T2 hyperintense lesions with little to no enhancement and may have calcifications. These slow-growing gliomas are thought to originate from multipotent glial progenitor cells in the central canal.[7] The eccentric or subpial growth pattern of subependymomas produces steep swelling of the spinal cord, which can give the appearance of the "bamboo leaf sign" on sagittal imaging[18,19] (Fig. 4).

Astrocytoma

Spinal astrocytomas account for approximately one-third of primary spinal cord tumors in adults, two-thirds of those in adolescents, and 90% of

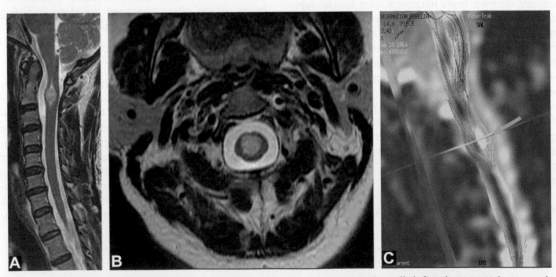

Fig. 1. Sagittal (A) and axial (B) T2WI images show a hyperintense, expansile well-defined, concentric mass originating from the central canal related to an ependymoma. Sagittal DTI image (C) shows the ependymoma is displacing adjacent tissues (arrow). (Courtesy of L Tanenbaum, MD, New York, New York.)

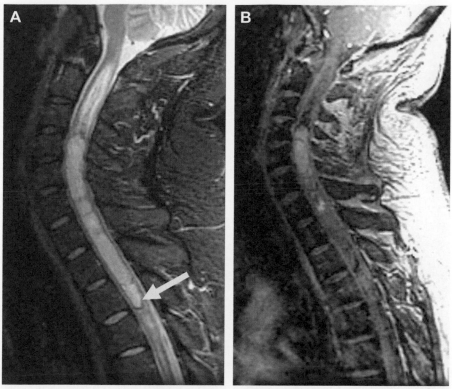

Fig. 2. Sagittal STIR (*A*) image show an expansile mass with associated cysts and syrinx. A subtle hypointense hemosiderin "cap sign" is seen along the inferior margin (*arrow*). Sagittal postcontrast T1WI (*B*) shows intense enhancement of the WHO grade 2 ependymoma.

those in children aged younger than 10 years.[20] They have a 2:3 female:male ratio and present during the third to fifth decades.[7] Spinal astrocytomas include pilocytic astrocytoma (WHO grade 1), accounting for 11% of pediatric spinal tumors and less that 1% of adult spinal tumors, diffuse astrocytoma (WHO grade 2), anaplastic astrocytoma (WHO grade 3), and glioblastoma (WHO grade 4).[21] The new WHO classification system for CNS tumors includes an integrated histologic-molecular diagnosis for astrocytomas.[9] Some common mutations observed in cranial astrocytomas are also noted in spinal astrocytomas, including mutations in the p16 gene, PTEN, BRAF, p53, and the replication independent histone 3 variant H3.3 gene. Specifically, p53 mutations are frequent in spinal cord astrocytomas,[22,23] and the spinal cord is one of the more common locations for astrocytomas mutated by histone H3 on lysine 27 (H3K27) in adults (Fig. 5). Spinal astrocytomas may be associated with neurofibromatosis type 1.

Spinal astrocytomas are typically thoracic in location and can vary in morphology from circumscribed to diffuse or infiltrative. In general, the circumscribed astrocytomas tend to be lower grade (WHO grades 1–3) and manifest in younger patients, often with well-defined enhancing masses.[18] Pilocytic astrocytomas (WHO grade 1), for example, are circumscribed gliomas, comprising 85% of pediatric astrocytomas, that tend to displace rather than infiltrate surrounding tissues. These lesions can enhance intensely and have cystic or hemorrhagic components. Pilomyxoid astrocytoma is a rare pediatric (often in children aged younger than 4 years) low-grade neoplasm that usually presents in the suprasellar/hypothalamic region but has been reported throughout the neuroaxis. Pilomyxoid astrocytomas have unique histologic features, high rato of CSF dissemination, and more aggressive behavior. On MR imaging, they may have solid and cystic components with T2 hyperintensity, diffusion hypointensity, and variable enhancement[24] (Fig. 6). The histology of these tumors reflects the imaging because there are compact fascicular regions with piloid processes and loose microcystic regions with pools of myxoid material,[25] which correlate with elevated water content and apparent diffusion coefficient (ADC) values.

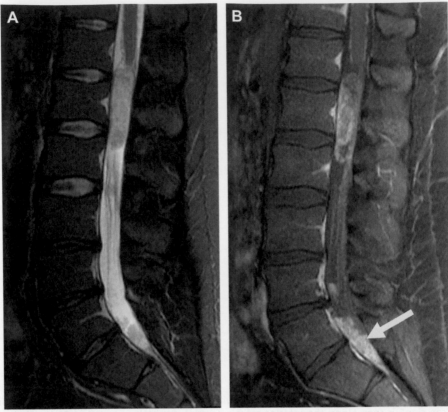

Fig. 3. Sagittal STIR (*A*) image shows a hyperintense mass of the filum terminale, with the involvement of the cauda equina nerve roots related to a myxopapillary ependymoma (WHO grade 2). Sagittal postcontrast T1WI (*B*) shows marked enhancement of the lesion. Note the intradural metastatic disease within the inferior thecal sac (*arrow*). Cranial spread of metastatic disease may also be seen with myxopapillary ependymoma.

These low-grade tumors can sometimes manifest with entire spinal cord (holocord) involvement, leptomeningeal dissemination, or fluorodeoxyglucose hypermetabolism, mimicking a more aggressive high-grade neoplasm.

Infiltrative astrocytomas tend to be higher grade (WHO grades 2–4) and occur in older patients.[18] Diffuse midline glioma, H3K27M-altered, is a grade 4 astrocytoma that can affect the spinal cord and occurs typically in children or young adults (see Fig. 5). H3K27M-altered spinal astrocytomas have a worse prognosis compared with nonmutated grade 4 spinal astrocytomas, with a 5-year median survival of only 14%.

The diagnosis of infiltrative astrocytomas can be challenging because the imaging may overlap with tumor mimics such as neuromyelitis optica spectrum disorder and neurosarcoidosis. Astrocytomas eccentrically expand the spinal cord and demonstrate variable enhancement patterns from nonenhancing to homogeneously or heterogeneously enhancing (Fig. 7). Enhancement usually correlates with a higher tumor grade, lower rates

of 5-year survival and is often used as a marker of malignant degeneration (Fig. 8). Infiltrative astrocytomas seem T1 hypointense to isointense and T2 hyperintense with ill-defined boundaries and peritumoral edema.

Hemangioblastoma

Hemangioblastoma is the third most common primary spinal cord neoplasm, occurring in less than 10% of cases.[12] Most cerebellar and spinal hemangioblastomas are sporadic and manifest in middle-aged adults (mean age of 48 years).[26] The familial cases associated with von Hippel–Lindau syndrome comprise approximately 25% of cases, presenting at a younger age with multiple hemangioblastomas.[27] This WHO grade 1 mesenchymal nonneuroepithelial tumor is composed of neoplastic stromal cells; it originates from primitive embryonic multipotent stem cells (hemangioblasts) and often demonstrates mutations of the von Hippel–Lindau tumor suppressor gene on chromosome 3.[25]

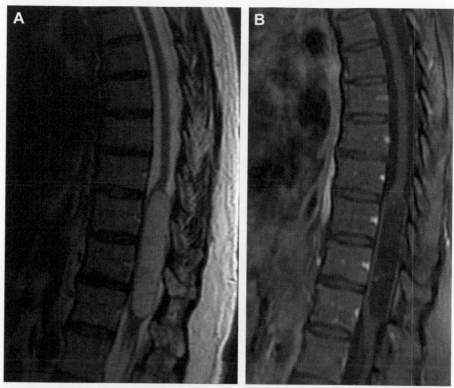

Fig. 4. Sagittal T2WI (*A*) image shows a hyperintense mass with an eccentric growth pattern that produces steep swelling of the spinal cord known as the "bamboo leaf sign." Sagittal postcontrast T1WI (*B*) image with fat-saturation shows no enhancement, typical of subependymoma.

Hemangioblastomas are mainly located at thoracic and cervical levels.[28] These tumors may have different morphologies: (1) intramedullary location with syringomyelia (~40%) and cord enlargement, (2) cord surface with exophytic growth and little reaction in the adjacent cord (snowman sign on contrast-enhanced images), or (3) exclusively extramedullary.[28,29] Posterior intramedullary location near the surface of the spinal cord predominates.[29] On MR imaging, hemangioblastomas are typically T1 isointense to hypointense and T2 isointense to hyperintense and exhibit marked enhancement due to hypervascularity. Smaller lesions show homogeneous enhancement, whereas large lesions enhance heterogeneously.[30] Vascular flow-voids may be seen, especially in tumors greater than 15 mm[28,30] (**Fig. 9**). Extensive cord edema and syringohydromyelia out of proportion to lesion size, possibly related to arteriovenous shunting or venous congestion, are helpful imaging clues.[28] Tumoral fluid secretion from leaky vessels causes syringomyelia or a "cyst with nodule" appearance in more than 50% of cases and often contributes to clinical symptoms (**Fig. 10**). Intramedullary and intratumoral hemorrhage may result in acute clinical presentations.[27]

Ganglioglioma/Gangliocytoma

Ganglioglioma/gangliocytoma is a rare WHO grade 1 tumor of neuronal origin, originating from the central gray matter. Spinal cord ganglioglioma has been observed in a wide age range of patients with most in children or young adults (mean age of 12 years). These lesions have indolent growth with long tumor length at presentation. Patients typically present with progressive myelopathy, in addition to other neurologic deficits related to location of the lesion. MR imaging demonstrates a circumscribed solid or mixed solid and cystic mass spanning a long segment of the cord with T1 hypointensity, T2 hyperintensity, and variable enhancement. Adjacent cord edema and syringomyelia and peritumoral cysts may be present in addition to reactive scoliosis[31] (**Fig. 11**).

CNS Lymphoma

Extranodal lymphoma of the spine is more often secondary and extradural in origin and location. Primary lymphoma of the spinal cord accounts for only 1% of primary CNS lymphoma (diffuse large B-cell) and usually manifests in middle-aged or older adults.[32] The most common

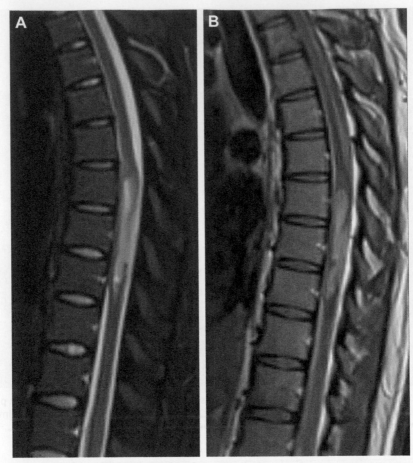

Fig. 5. Sagittal STIR (*A*) image shows an expansile hyperintense mass spanning multiple vertebral levels. Sagittal postcontrast T1WI (*B*) image shows marked enhancement of the mass with ill-defined margins. Pathology revealed a diffuse midline glioma H3K27M-altered.

intramedullary location is the cervical spinal cord, with a solitary lesion in most patients. Intramedullary lymphoma may also be due to the invasion of leptomeningeal disease.[33]

The hypercellularity of lymphoma results in hyperattenuation on CT, hypointensity on T2WI and ADC mapping, and hypermetabolism on fluorodeoxyglucose positron emission tomography (18F-FDG PET; Fig. 12). On MR imaging, intramedullary lymphoma seems as poorly circumscribed, T1 isointense, T2 hypointense/isointense lesions with variable enhancement. There is usually no accompanying cystic or hemorrhagic component, distinguishing it from glial tumors. Concurrent enhancing lesions suggestive of CNS lymphoma on cranial MR imaging may be present.

Melanocytic Tumors

Primary melanocytic tumors include benign or malignant and focal or diffuse entities such as meningeal melanocytoma, melanoma, melanocytosis,

and melanomatosis. These lesions originate from melanocytes, which are nonneuroepithelial cells originating in the neural crest. Spinal meningeal melanocytoma or melanoma is usually homogeneously enhancing, with T1 isointensity to hyperintensity and T2 isointensity to hypointensity, depending on the melanin content[34,35] (Fig. 13).

METASTASES

Intramedullary metastases from non-CNS primaries are rare with a reported frequency of 0.9% to 2.1% on autopsy series.[36] The majority are from a lung primary (50%), followed by breast primary.[37] These may occur secondary to hematogenous dissemination, retrograde venous spread, perineural lymphatic spread, or direct invasion.[37] Most spinal cord metastases are solitary and often localized to the thoracic or cervical spinal cord (80%).[37]

Intramedullary metastases are T1 isointense and T2 hyperintense, often with extensive

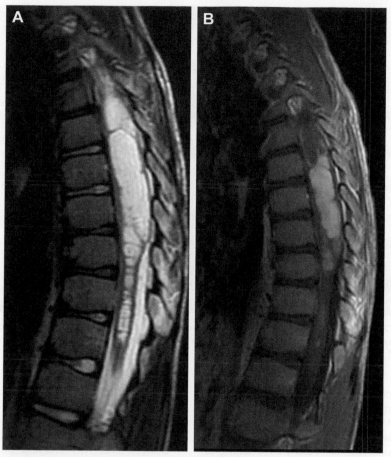

Fig. 6. Sagittal T2WI (*A*) image shows an expansile, cystic, hyperintense mass related to a pilomyxoid astrocytoma. Sagittal postcontrast T1WI (*B*) image shows marked enhancement.

surrounding edema (mean 4.5 segments) and prominent contrast enhancement.[37] Valuable MR imaging findings are the rim and flame signs. The rim sign denotes thin peripheral enhancement with less intense central enhancement, occurring more commonly in metastasis (33%) compared with other cord tumors (3%).[38] The flame sign describes ill-defined tapering enhancement at the rostral and caudal aspects of the lesion and is more common in metastasis (30%) than other cord tumors (3%)[38] (**Fig. 14**). Intramedullary metastases are typically hypermetabolic on 18F-FDG PET (**Fig. 15**).

Cystic Lesions

Spinal cystic lesions may be associated with neoplasms or can be congenital in origin. There are various developmental intradural spinal cysts including enterogenous cysts, teratomatous cysts, arachnoid cysts, neurenteric cysts, foregut cysts, and bronchogenic cysts. Spinal ependymal

cyst is a rare intramedullary lesion that has the potential to expand secondary to secretion of fluid into the cyst cavity. The local mass effect may lead to neurologic deficits.[39] It can be challenging to distinguish between various intramedullary cystic lesions based solely on MR imaging findings. Ependymal cyst borders are smooth and well defined. These typically ventrally located lesions are isointense to CSF on T1WI and T2WI without peripheral enhancement. Unlike epidermoid cysts, ependymal cysts will show fluid signal intensity on diffusion weighted imaging (DWI; **Fig. 16**).

ADVANCED IMAGING OF SPINAL CORD TUMORS

Primary spinal tumor intratumoral heterogeneity may lead to either underestimating or overestimating the amount of tumor tissue on MR imaging.[40] Molecular imaging with positron emission tomography of primary or secondary CNS spinal tumors

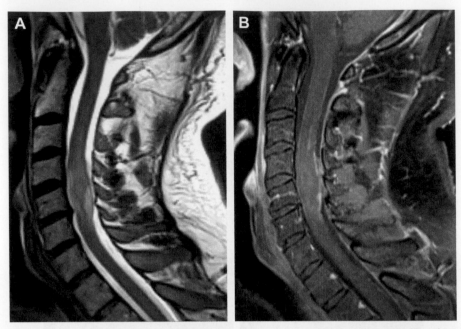

Fig. 7. Sagittal T2WI (A) image shows an expansile hyperintense mass eccentrically expanding the spinal cord. Sagittal postcontrast T1WI (B) image with fat-saturation shows mild, feathery enhancement in this WHO grade 2 astrocytoma.

may be performed to identify metabolically active tumor compartments, differentiation of viable tumor tissue from necrosis, and prediction of treatment response by measurement of tumor perfusion or ischemia. 18F-FDG-PET imaging is useful in evaluating tumor progression and identifying the most metabolically active components in spinal cord tumors[41] (see Fig. 15). Generally, 18F-FDG-PET is used to predict the growth rate of a neoplasm. Correlation with histologic malignancy in spinal gliomas has also been reported.[42]

Conventional MR imaging primarily provides anatomic information on spinal cord tumors and their relationship to surrounding structures.

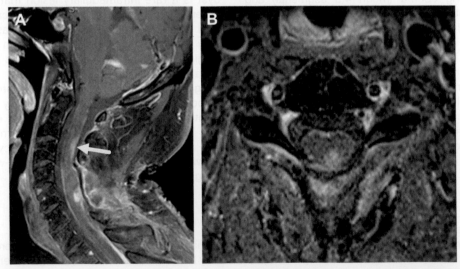

Fig. 8. Sagittal (A) and axial (B) postcontrast T1WI images with fat-saturation show marked enhancement of the intramedullary mass with CSF dissemination (arrow), in same patient from Fig. 7, which degenerated to WHO grade 4.

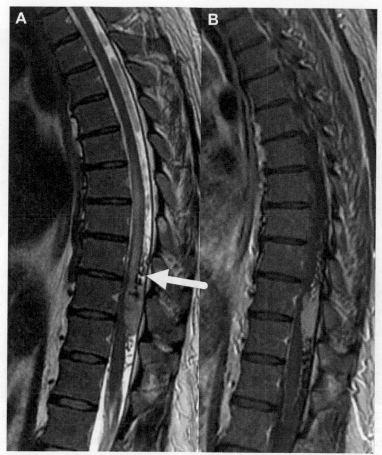

Fig. 9. Sagittal T2WI (*A*) image shows an expansile mildly hyperintense mass along the dorsal surface of the thoracic spinal cord, with prominent vascular flow voids (*arrow*). Sagittal postcontrast T1WI (*B*) image shows marked enhancement of this hemangioblastoma.

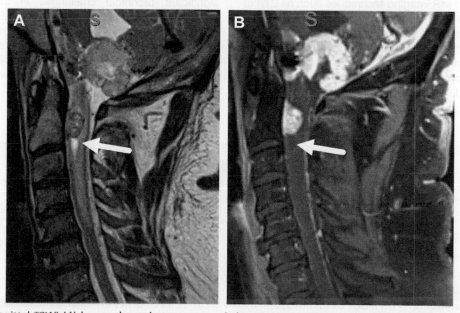

Fig. 10. Sagittal T2WI (*A*) image shows heterogeneously hypointense masses at the C2 level and in the inferior cerebellar vermis. Sagittal postcontrast T1WI (*B*) image with fat-saturation reveals an intensely enhancing mural nodule along the pial surface in this hemangioblastoma with a "cyst and mural nodule" appearance (*arrow*).

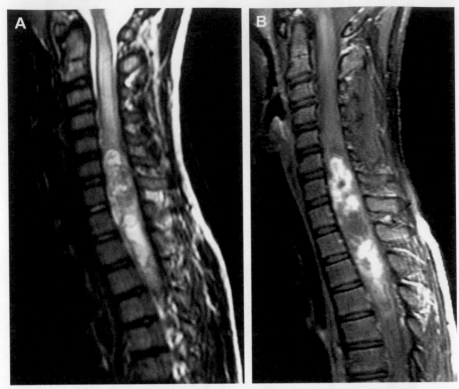

Fig. 11. Sagittal T2WI image (*A*) shows an expansile heterogeneously hyperintense mass expanding the cervical spinal cord with surrounding edema and areas of cystic change. Sagittal T1WI post-contrast image (*B*) reveals heterogenous enhancement of this intramedullary tumor, pathologically proven to be a ganglioglioma. (*Courtesy of* Susan Blaser, MD).

Advanced MR imaging techniques such as DWI or diffusion tensor imaging (DTI) may be performed to assess tumor's cellularity and its impact on longitudinal white matter tracts (tractography), respectively. MR perfusion imaging can provide information on tumoral vascularity. However, advanced MR imaging techniques encounter

significant technical challenges in the spinal cord. The small size of the spinal cord requires the use of small voxel sizes (higher matrix) for spatial resolution that decreases the signal-to-noise ratio.[43] Image degradation can be caused by CSF flow/pulsation, breathing, swallowing, and susceptibility artifact from the vertebral

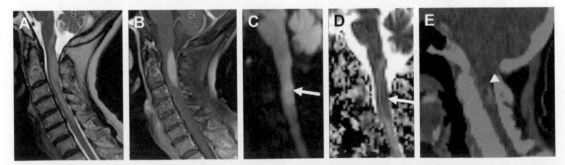

Fig. 12. Sagittal T2WI (*A*) image shows an expansile mass at the C2 level, with surrounding edema. Sagittal post-contrast T1WI (*B*) image with fat-saturation reveals an intensely enhancing mass in the dorsal cord, reflecting intramedullary lymphoma. Sagittal DTI TRACE (*C*) and ADC (*D*) reveal hyperintensity and hypointensity, respectively (*arrows*). Sagittal FDG PET-CT (*E*) demonstrates avid tracer uptake (*arrowhead*).

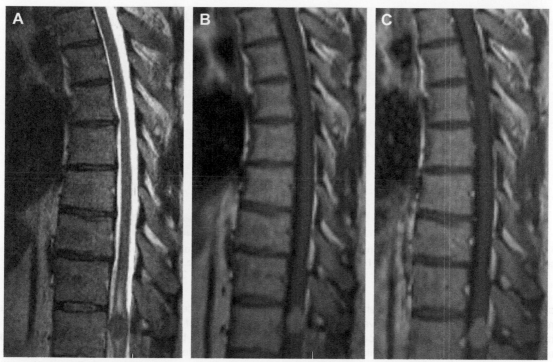

Fig. 13. Sagittal T2WI (*A*) image reveals an intramedullary, circumscribed hypointense lesion in the thoracic spinal cord with mild edema. Sagittal T1WI (*B*) and postcontrast T1WI (*C*) images show that this melanocytoma is T1 hyperintense with mild enhancement.

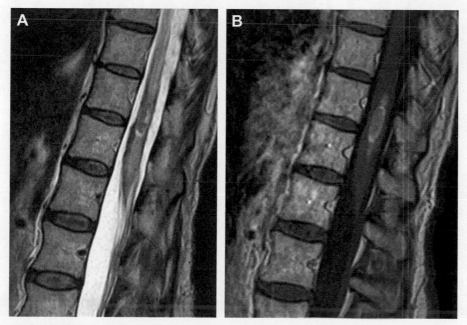

Fig. 14. Sagittal T2WI (*A*) image shows an intramedullary heterogeneously hypointense lesion in the conus medullaris with surrounding edema. Sagittal postcontrast T1WI (*B*) image illustrates the rim and flame signs of this intramedullary metastasis from breast cancer.

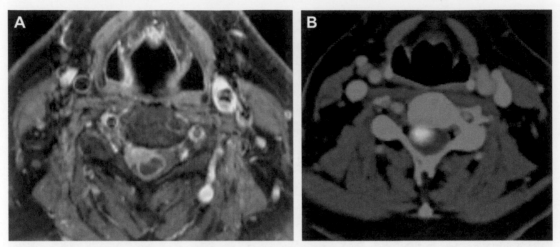

Fig. 15. Axial postcontrast T1WI (*A*) image shows an intramedullary cystic and solid metastasis from prostate cancer. Axial FDG PET (*B*) image reveals hypermetabolism in the solid nodule.

column. Local field inhomogeneities may also reduce image resolution by preventing efficient rephasing of proton spins, typically seen with echoplanar DWI/DTI. These technical issues also limit acquisition of nuclear magnetic resonance (NMR) spectra with adequate signal-to-noise ratio for magnetic resonance spectroscopy of spinal cord lesions. As such, there are limited data using

such advanced imaging techniques for the assessment of pathologic processes.

DWI/DTI is based on the Brownian motion of water molecules (isotropic). In the CNS, water motion is restricted by axonal myelin sheaths with relative preference of water movement along the axon (anisotropy) and limited perpendicular to the axon length.

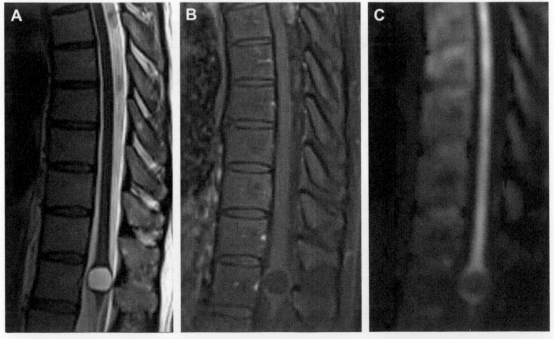

Fig. 16. Sagittal T2WI (*A*) image reveals a circumscribed, intramedullary hyperintense lesion in the conus medullaris without edema. Sagittal postcontrast T1WI (*B*) image shows no enhancement of this ependymal cyst (ventriculus terminalis). Sagittal DTI TRACE (*C*) image shows signal intensity similar to that of CSF.

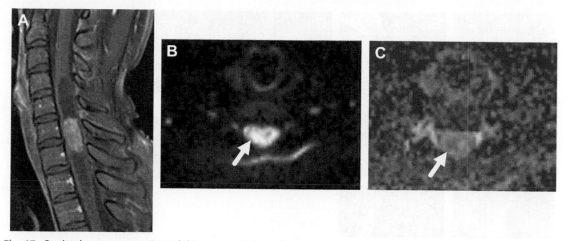

Fig. 17. Sagittal postcontrast T1WI (*A*) image with fat-saturation demonstrates an expansile intramedullary lesion with a discrete enhancing nodule. Axial DTI TRACE shows hyperintensity (*B*) and ADC (*C*) hypointensity (*arrows*) in the enhancing nodule of an ependymoma.

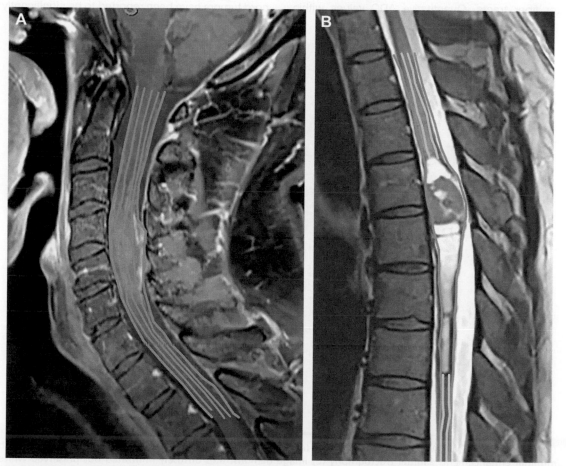

Fig. 18. DTI tractography of spinal cord astrocytoma (*A*) shows encasement of fibers. In an ependymoma (*B*), DTI tractography exhibits displaced fibers.

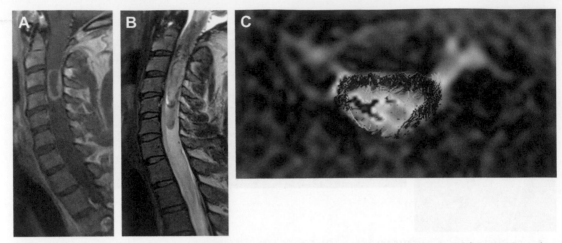

Fig. 19. Sagittal postcontrast T1WI (*A*) and T2WI (*B*) images show a rim-enhancing mass with extensive edema within the cord. Axial tractography (*C*) image demonstrates displaced white matter tracts around the lesion, consistent with expected behavior of ependymoma. (*Courtesy of* M Mossa-Basha, MD, Seattle, Washington.)

DTI metrics (eg, ADC, fractional anisotropy [FA], radial diffusivity, axial diffusivity) can quantitatively assess the water movement along the white matter fiber tracts. Quantitative ADC values within intramedullary tumors can be variable[44] with low values suggesting hypercellularity (Fig. 17). The FA values of most of enhancing or nonenhancing cord tumors have been reported to be significantly

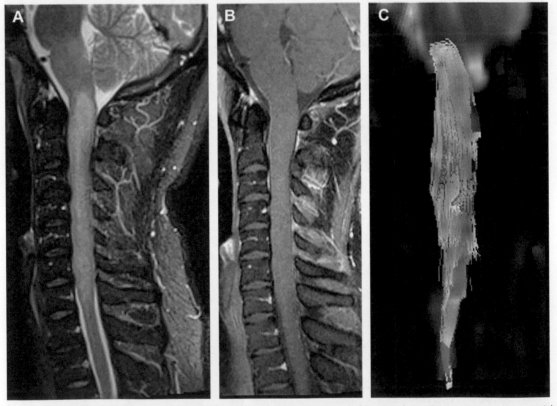

Fig. 20. Sagittal T2WI (*A*) and postcontrast T1WI (*B*) images show an infiltrative hyperintense astrocytoma with minimal enhancement. Sagittal tractography (*C*) image demonstrates diffusely infiltrated but preserved white matter fibers; therefore, the lesion was amenable to biopsy rather than resection, followed by radiation. (*Courtesy of* V Shah, MD, San Francisco, California.)

decreased compared with normal or reference regions, which suggests the destruction of normal fiber structure or tumor infiltrative changes. Conversely, FA may be increased within intramedullary tumors, which may relate to the infiltrative growth of astrocytoma cells along fibers and/or to the tumor encompassing the fiber tracts.[44] An early study of DTI in spinal cord tumors showed FA values to be similar for astrocytomas, ependymomas, and metastases but different for hemangioblastomas.[45] The FA map is useful in detecting the extent of a spinal cord tumor[46,47] and distinguishing it from the surrounding edema.

Spinal cord fiber tracts are oriented craniocaudally (descending) or caudocranially (ascending).

The directional component of DTI can be used to generate 3-dimensional fiber tractography, which can provide noninvasive visual assessment of the integrity of white matter fibers in vivo, in relation to the spinal cord tumors.[45–55] Preoperative DTI tractography can demonstrate the relationship between white matter fibers and spinal cord tumors, aiding surgical planning. Displacement of white matter fibers is suggestive of benignity and increased possibility of complete resection[47–49,53,54,56] (Fig. 18). Because spinal ependymomas have only a slight likelihood of infiltrating the adjacent neural tissue, and have a discrete capsule forming a cleavage plane between the tumor and the spinal cord, the fibers on tractography

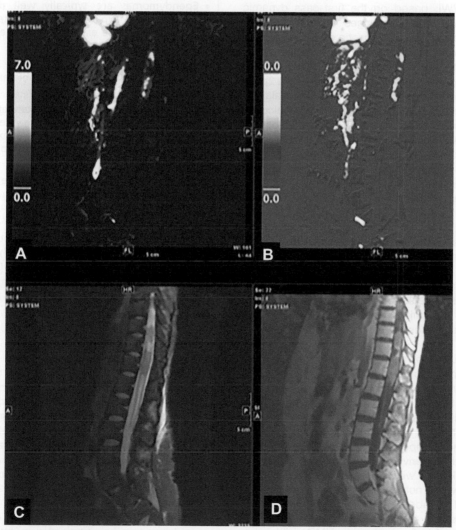

Fig. 21. (A) Sagittal DCE demonstrates elevated plasma volume (Vp) in the intramedullary enhancing lesion. Vp correlates with BV. (B) Sagittal DCE shows elevated K-trans in the intramedullary mass, reflecting increased vascular permeability in the intramedullary breast cancer metastasis. Sagittal STIR (C) and postcontrast T1WI (D) demonstrate hypointensity and heterogeneous enhancement of the intramedullary lesion, respectively. DCE, dynamic contrast enhancing imaging. (Courtesy of H Stambuk, MD, New York, New York.)

tend to be displaced[45] (Fig. 19). Spinal astrocytomas can demonstrate more aggressive behavior and may infiltrate or encase the white matter tracts.[45] The low-grade fibrillary or pilocytic astrocytomas tend to displace rather than infiltrate the cord[47,48,50–54,56,57] (Fig. 20). In addition to white matter fiber displacement and encasement by tumor, fibers may also cross the tumor.[54] An important clinical application of DTI tractography is for surgical guidance, to obtain safer maximal resection of spinal cord tumors with the preservation of neurologic function.[47,48,53]

Advanced techniques such as MR perfusion weighted imaging (PWI) can be used to evaluate the hemodynamic characteristics of spinal cord tumors.[44,58,59] With dynamic susceptibility contrast-PWI, based on the first-pass dynamic $T2^*$ signal intensity changes after intravenous bolus injection of paramagnetic contrast material, the relative blood volume (BV) ratio may be derived. Because it is common for spinal cord tumors to involve the transverse extent of the spinal cord, it is difficult to get the BV in the contralateral normal-appearing cord as a reference to calculate the relative BV ratio. Therefore, it is suggested that relative BV be used as a qualitative measurement tool, and the peak height and percentage of signal intensity recovery, which are independent of rBV algorithms, be used for quantitative perfusion assessment.[60] Preliminary studies have found both quantitative peak height and qualitative BV map can demonstrate the increased perfusion within the nonenhancing and enhancing spinal cord tumors.[44,58,59] The literature is sparse regarding dynamic contrast-enhanced MR imaging (evaluation of temporal delivery and washout of contrast agents into and out of the tumor, reflecting the microvascular distribution within the tissue) assessment of spinal cord tumors (Fig. 21).

Few studies of magnetic resonance spectroscopy of spinal cord lesions have been performed. A case series of 14 patients with a spectrum of spinal cord lesions demonstrated most benign lesions and tumors showed lipid signals in their 1H spectra. Mobile lipids were frequently encountered in the MR spectra of actively growing tumors and could be derived from membrane or myelin-lipid breakdown without cell necrosis.[61] Elevated choline was noted in tumors, representing increased membrane synthesis of rapidly proliferating cells and the breakdown of NMR-invisible phosphatidylcholine, releasing NMR-visible cholines in viable tumor irrespective of malignancy.[62] In ependymomas, glycine may be elevated without choline.[62,63] Metastases show high lipid signals and enhanced choline.[62,64]

SUMMARY

Spinal cord tumors have varied imaging appearances and clinical features, which are affected by histology and molecular status. Certain MR imaging characteristics can help distinguish spinal cord tumors. Continued development of advanced imaging techniques hold great promise not only for the identification of spinal cord neoplasms but also for treatment planning and response.

CLINICS CARE POINTS

- Ependymomas are typically well defined, concentrically expansile T2 hyperintense lesions with intense enhancement. They often have hemorrhage and cysts.

- Astrocytomas are classically diffusely infiltrative expansile masses with variable enhancement patterns.

- Hemangioblastomas are characterized by an avidly enhancing nodule along the dorsal subpial spinal cord, with a cyst and extensive edema. When large, vascular flow voids may be identified.

- Metastatic intramedullary tumors are characterized by marked enhancement and extensive surrounding edema. Helpful imaging signs include the rim and flame signs.

- Diffusion tractography may demonstrate displacement of the fibers in ependymomas and infiltration of fibers in astrocytoma.

DISCLOSURE

The authors have nothing to disclose.

REFERENCES

1. Duong LM, McCarthy BJ, McLendon RE, et al. Descriptive epidemiology of malignant and nonmalignant primary spinal cord, spinal meninges, and cauda equina tumors, United States, 2004-2007. Cancer 2012;118(17):4220–7.

2. Grimm S, Chamberlain MC. Adult primary spinal cord tumors. Expert Rev Neurother 2009;9(10): 1487–95.

3. Tobin MK, Geraghty JR, Engelhard HH, et al. Intramedullary spinal cord tumors: a review of current and future treatment strategies. Neurosurg Focus 2015;39(2):E14.

4. Kotecha R, Mehta MP, Chang EL, et al. Updates in the management of intradural spinal cord tumors:

a radiation oncology focus. Neuro Oncol 2019;21(6): 707–18.

5. Rossi A, Gandolfo C, Morana G, et al. Tumors of the spine in children. Neuroimaging Clin N Am 2007; 17(1):17–35.

6. Merhemic Z, Stosic-Opincal T, Thurnher MM. Neuroimaging of Spinal Tumors. Magn Reson Imag Clin N Am 2016;24(3):563–79.

7. Ottenhausen M, Ntoulias G, Bodhinayake I, et al. Intradural spinal tumors in adults-update on management and outcome. Neurosurg Rev 2019;42(2): 371–88.

8. Ellison DW, Aldape KD, Capper D, et al. cIMPACT-NOW update 7: advancing the molecular classification of ependymal tumors. Brain Pathol 2020;30(5): 863–6.

9. Louis DN, Perry A, Wesseling P, et al. The 2021 WHO Classification of Tumors of the Central Nervous System: a summary. Neuro Oncol 2021;23(8):1231–51.

10. Swanson AA, Raghunathan A, Jenkins RB, et al. Spinal Cord Ependymomas With MYCN Amplification Show Aggressive Clinical Behavior. J Neuropathol Exp Neurol 2019;78(9):791–7.

11. Kim DH, Kim JH, Choi SH, et al. Differentiation between intramedullary spinal ependymoma and astrocytoma: comparative MRI analysis. Clin Radiol 2014;69(1):29–35.

12. Koeller KK, Rosenblum RS, Morrison AL. Neoplasms of the spinal cord and filum terminale: radiologic-pathologic correlation. Radiographics 2000;20(6): 1721–49.

13. Kobayashi K, Ando K, Kato F, et al. MRI Characteristics of Spinal Ependymoma in WHO Grade II: A Review of 59 Cases. Spine 2018;43(9):E525–30.

14. Kobayashi K, Ando K, Kato F, et al. Variety of preoperative MRI changes in spinal cord ependymoma of WHO grade II: a case series. Eur Spine J 2019; 28(2):426–33.

15. Sun B, Wang C, Wang J, et al. MRI features of intramedullary spinal cord ependymomas. J Neuroimaging 2003;13(4):346–51.

16. Dauleac C, Messerer R, Obadia-Andre N, et al. Cysts associated with intramedullary ependymomas of the spinal cord: clinical, MRI and oncological features. J Neuro Oncol 2019;144(2):385–91.

17. Frazier AA. Myxopapillary Ependymoma. Radiographics 2019;39(2):467.

18. Shih RY, Koeller KK. Intramedullary Masses of the Spinal Cord: Radiologic-Pathologic Correlation. Radiographics 2020;40(4):1125–45.

19. Toi H, Ogawa Y, Kinoshita K, et al. Bamboo Leaf Sign as a Sensitive Magnetic Resonance Imaging Finding in Spinal Subependymoma: Case Report and Literature Review. Case Rep Neurol Med 2016;2016:9108641.

20. Ostrom QT, Gittleman H, Farah P, et al. CBTRUS statistical report: Primary brain and central nervous system tumors diagnosed in the United States in 2006-2010. Neuro Oncol 2013;15(Suppl 2):ii1–56.

21. Nadkarni TD, Rekate HL. Pediatric intramedullary spinal cord tumors. Critical review of the literature. Childs Nerv Syst 1999;15(1):17–28.

22. Yanamadala V, Koffie RM, Shankar GM, et al. Spinal cord glioblastoma: 25years of experience from a single institution. J Clin Neurosci 2016;27:138–41.

23. Nagaishi M, Yokoo H, Nobusawa S, et al. A distinctive pediatric case of low-grade glioma with extensive expression of CD34. Brain Tumor Pathol 2016;33(1):71–4.

24. Garber ST, Bollo RJ, Riva-Cambrin JK. Pediatric spinal pilomyxoid astrocytoma. J Neurosurg Pediatr 2013;12(5):511–6.

25. Perry A, Rosenblum MK. Central nervous system. Amsterdam, the Netherlands: Elsevier; 2018.

26. Westwick HJ, Giguere JF, Shamji MF. Incidence and Prognosis of Spinal Hemangioblastoma: A Surveillance Epidemiology and End Results Study. Neuroepidemiology 2016;46(1):14–23.

27. Kiyofuji S, Graffeo CS, Yokoyama M, et al. Intramedullary and intratumoral hemorrhage in spinal hemangioblastoma: Case report and review of literature. Surg Neurol Int 2018;9:250.

28. Baker KB, Moran CJ, Wippold FJ 2nd, et al. MR imaging of spinal hemangioblastoma. AJR American journal of roentgenology 2000;174(2):377–82.

29. Imagama S, Ito Z, Wakao N, et al. Differentiation of localization of spinal hemangioblastomas based on imaging and pathological findings. Eur Spine J 2011;20(8):1377–84.

30. Chu BC, Terae S, Hida K, et al. MR findings in spinal hemangioblastoma: correlation with symptoms and with angiographic and surgical findings. AJNR American journal of neuroradiology 2001;22(1): 206–17.

31. Patel U, Pinto RS, Miller DC, et al. MR of spinal cord ganglioglioma. AJNR American journal of neuroradiology 1998;19(5):879 87.

32. Koeller KK, Shih RY. Extranodal Lymphoma of the Central Nervous System and Spine. Radiol Clin North Am 2016;54(4):649–71.

33. Haque S, Law M, Abrey LE, et al. Imaging of lymphoma of the central nervous system, spine, and orbit. Radiol Clin North Am 2008;46(2):339–61, ix.

34. Yang C, Fang J, Li G, et al. Spinal meningeal melanocytomas: clinical manifestations, radiological and pathological characteristics, and surgical outcomes. J Neuro Oncol 2016;127(2):279–86.

35. Huang X, Pan X, Huang H, et al. Multiple spinal cord melanoma: case report with emphasis on the difficult preoperative diagnosis. Turk Neurosurg 2013;23(4): 534–8.

36. Costigan DA, Winkelman MD. Intramedullary spinal cord metastasis. A clinicopathological study of 13 cases. J Neurosurg 1985;62(2):227–33.

37. Rykken JB, Diehn FE, Hunt CH, et al. Intramedullary spinal cord metastases: MRI and relevant clinical features from a 13-year institutional case series. AJNR American journal of neuroradiology 2013; 34(10):2043–9.

38. Rykken JB, Diehn FE, Hunt CH, et al. Rim and flame signs: postgadolinium MRI findings specific for non-CNS intramedullary spinal cord metastases. AJNR American journal of neuroradiology 2013;34(4): 908–15.

39. Yang T, Wu L, Deng X, et al. Clinical characteristics and surgical outcomes of spinal intramedullary ependymal cysts. Acta Neurochir 2014;156(2): 269–75.

40. Levivier M, Becerra A, De Witte O, et al. Radiation necrosis or recurrence. J Neurosurg 1996;84(1): 148–9.

41. ASPA. Bone Health and Osteoporosis: A Report of the Surgeon General 2004. Available at: http://www. surgeongeneral.gov/library/reports/bonehealth/ suggested_citation.html. Accessed November 25, 2013.

42. Wilmshurst JM, Barrington SF, Pritchard D, et al. Positron emission tomography in imaging spinal cord tumors. J Child Neurol 2000;15(7):465–72.

43. Maier SE, Mamata H. Diffusion tensor imaging of the spinal cord. Ann N Y Acad Sci 2005;1064:50–60.

44. Liu X, Tian W, Kolar B, et al. Advanced MR diffusion tensor imaging and perfusion weighted imaging of intramedullary tumors and tumor like lesions in the cervicomedullary junction region and the cervical spinal cord. J Neuro Oncol 2014;116(3):559–66.

45. Ducreux D, Lepeintre JF, Fillard P, et al. MR diffusion tensor imaging and fiber tracking in 5 spinal cord astrocytomas. AJNR American journal of neuroradiology 2006;27(1):214–6.

46. Ducreux D, Fillard P, Facon D, et al. Diffusion tensor magnetic resonance imaging and fiber tracking in spinal cord lesions: current and future indications. Neuroimaging Clin N Am 2007;17(1):137–47.

47. Landi A, Palmarini V, D'Elia A, et al. Magnetic resonance diffusion tensor imaging and fiber-tracking diffusion tensor tractography in the management of spinal astrocytomas. World J Clin Cases 2016;4(1): 1–4.

48. Mechtler LL, Nandigam K. Spinal cord tumors: new views and future directions. Neurol Clin 2013;31(1): 241–68.

49. Bloomer CW, Ackerman A, Bhatia RG. Imaging for spine tumors and new applications. Top Magn Reson Imaging 2006;17(2):69–87.

50. Baruah D, Chandra T, Bajaj M, et al. A simplified algorithm for diagnosis of spinal cord lesions. Curr Probl Diagn Radiol 2015;44(3):256–66.

51. Rajasekaran S, Kanna RM, Shetty AP. Diffusion tensor imaging of the spinal cord and its clinical applications. The Journal of bone and joint surgery British 2012;94(8):1024–31.

52. Thurnher MM, Law M. Diffusion-weighted imaging, diffusion-tensor imaging, and fiber tractography of the spinal cord. Magn Reson Imag Clin N Am 2009;17(2):225–44.

53. Choudhri AF, Whitehead MT, Klimo P Jr, et al. Diffusion tensor imaging to guide surgical planning in intramedullary spinal cord tumors in children. Neuroradiology 2014;56(2):169–74.

54. Setzer M, Murtagh RD, Murtagh FR, et al. Diffusion tensor imaging tractography in patients with intramedullary tumors: comparison with intraoperative findings and value for prediction of tumor resectability. J Neurosurg Spine 2010;13(3):371–80.

55. Phillips NS, Sanford RA, Helton KJ, et al. Diffusion tensor imaging of intraaxial tumors at the cervicomedullary and pontomedullary junctions. Report of two cases. J Neurosurg 2005;103(6 Suppl):557–62.

56. Vargas MI, Delavelle J, Jlassi H, et al. Clinical applications of diffusion tensor tractography of the spinal cord. Neuroradiology 2008;50(1):25–9.

57. Martin AR, Aleksanderek I, Cohen-Adad J, et al. Translating state-of-the-art spinal cord MRI techniques to clinical use: A systematic review of clinical studies utilizing DTI, MT, MWF, MRS, and fMRI. NeuroImage Clinical 2016;10:192–238.

58. Liu X, Germin BI, Ekholm S. A case of cervical spinal cord glioblastoma diagnosed with MR diffusion tensor and perfusion imaging. J Neuroimaging 2011;21(3):292–6.

59. Liu X, Kolar B, Tian W, et al. MR perfusion-weighted imaging may help in differentiating between nonenhancing gliomas and nonneoplastic lesions in the cervicomedullary junction. J Magn Reson Imag 2011;34(1):196–202.

60. Liu X, Tian W, Chen H, et al. Advanced Neuroimaging in the Evaluation of Spinal Cord Tumors and Tumor Mimics: Diffusion Tensor and Perfusion-Weighted Imaging. Semin Ultrasound CT MR 2017; 38(2):163–75.

61. Kuesel AC, Donnelly SM, Halliday W, et al. Mobile lipids and metabolic heterogeneity of brain tumours as detectable by ex vivo 1H MR spectroscopy. NMR Biomed 1994;7(4):172–80.

62. Kim YG, Choi GH, Kim DH, et al. In vivo proton magnetic resonance spectroscopy of human spinal mass lesions. J Spinal Disord Tech 2004;17(5): 405–11.

63. Kinoshita Y, Yokota A. Absolute concentrations of metabolites in human brain tumors using in vitro proton magnetic resonance spectroscopy. NMR Biomed 1997;10(1):2–12.

64. Sijens PE, Knopp MV, Brunetti A, et al. 1H MR spectroscopy in patients with metastatic brain tumors: a multicenter study. Magn Reson Med 1995;33(6): 818–26.

Intradural Extramedullary Tumors and Associated Syndromes

Paulo Puac-Polanco, MD, MSc[a], Angela Guarnizo, MD[b],
Juan Pablo Cruz, MD[c], Francisco Rivas Rodriguez, MD[d],
Carlos H. Torres, MD, FRCPC, FCAR[a],*

KEYWORDS

• Spine • Spinal tumors • Intradural extramedullary • Cancer • MRI

KEY POINTS

- MR imaging is the modality of choice for detecting and evaluating intradural extramedullary spinal tumors.
- Most (70%–80%) of the intradural tumors are located within the intradural extramedullary compartment.
- Schwannomas and meningiomas are the most common intradural extramedullary spinal tumors.
- As the phenotype of patients with multiple schwannomas spans a continuum with significant overlapping features, a new classification has been proposed using the umbrella term schwannomatosis, along with the gene affected.
- Myxopapillary ependymoma is the most prevalent primary neoplasm of the conus medullaris and cauda equina.

INTRODUCTION

Most (70%–80%) of the intradural tumors are located within the intradural extramedullary compartment, and the most common tumors are schwannomas and meningiomas.[1] Other less common neoplasms include neurofibroma, solitary fibrous tumor (SFT), myxopapillary ependymoma (MPE), lymphoma, metastatic leptomeningeal disease, malignant peripheral nerve sheath tumor (MPNST), and paraganglioma. Patients usually present with gait ataxia, radicular pain, and motor and sensory deficits due to chronic compressive myelopathy or radiculopathy.

MR imaging is the modality of choice for detecting and evaluating intradural extramedullary spinal tumors due to its multiplanar capabilities and exquisite soft tissue contrast. The differential diagnosis is usually based on the tumor's location within the spinal canal and key imaging features on contrast-enhanced MR imaging. Age, gender, and clinical presentation are also important factors in determining the diagnosis. Ultimately, imaging is the key in narrowing the differential diagnosis and guiding patient management.

NORMAL ANATOMY AND IMAGING APPEARANCE OF THE SPINAL INTRADURAL SPACE

The three meningeal layers (dura mater, arachnoid layer, and pia mater) surrounding the cord are

[a] Department of Radiology, Radiation Oncology and Medical Physics, University of Ottawa, Box 232, General Campus Room 1466e, 501 Smyth Road, Ottawa, Ontario K1H 8L6, Canada; [b] Radiology- Department of Diagnostic Imaging, Hospital Universitario Fundación Santa Fe de Bogota, Carrera 7 # 117-15, 220246 Bogotá-Colombia; [c] Instituto de Neurocirugía Dr. Asenjo, Servicio de Neurorradiología Diagnóstica y Terapéutica, José Manuel Infante 553, Santiago, Providencia, Región Metropolitana, Chile; [d] Radiology, Division of Neuroradiology, University of Michigan, Michigan Medicine, C.S. Mott Children's Hospital, 1540 E Hospital Drive Rm 3-227, Ann Arbor, MI 48109-4252, USA

* Corresponding author.
E-mail address: catorres@toh.ca

Neuroimag Clin N Am 33 (2023) 407–422
https://doi.org/10.1016/j.nic.2023.03.002

developed around the 19th week of fetal life.[2] These meningeal layers create different compartments in the spinal canal that are useful for approaching spinal pathology. The intradural extramedullary space is located between the dura mater externally and the pia mater internally (Fig. 1). This compartment contains the arachnoid layer, cerebrospinal fluid (CSF), spinal nerves, and vessels.

The intradural extramedullary space follows the signal intensity of CSF on MR imaging: dark signal on T1-weighted images (WI) and bright signal on T2WI. However, the CSF signal intensity is frequently altered by CSF flow-related effects (time-of-flight artifacts and turbulent flow) that should not be mistaken for pathology (Fig. 2).[3]

The precise location of a spinal lesion has important implications for diagnosis and treatment. Given the mass effect and displacement of the cord, intradural lesions generally cause an enlargement of the subarachnoid space at the tumor margins, which helps distinguish them from lesions in the epidural space (Fig. 3).

IMAGING TECHNIQUE AND PROTOCOL

MR imaging is the modality of choice for evaluating spinal tumors, given its superior soft tissue contrast. In addition, MR imaging accurately depicts surrounding structures, such as vertebral column, neuroforamina, and spinal cord.

Computed tomography (CT) is reserved for preoperative delineation of bone anatomy, instrumentation planning, and to assess tumor calcification. Myelogram or CT myelogram in the era of MR imaging is restricted to a few conditions: MR imaging contraindication and postoperative spine cases with significant susceptibility artifacts arising from metallic hardware. MR imaging spine protocol includes sagittal T1, sagittal T2, and axial T2-weighted sequences. These sequences can be used as 2-dimensional (2D) or 3-dimensional (3D) acquisitions. Fat-suppressed T1WI post-contrast is vital in the evaluation of spinal tumors and allows to narrow the differential diagnosis and to exclude alternate conditions. Optional sequences include gradient-echo and diffusion-weighted imaging.

BENIGN NEOPLASMS
Meningioma

Spinal meningioma is one of the most common primary intradural extramedullary tumors and accounts for 20%–25% of tumors in this location.[4,5] Up to 80% of them are World Health Organization (WHO) grade 1. Higher tumor grades are associated with genetic alterations, such as telomerase reverse transcriptase (TERT) promoter mutation and CDKNA2A/B loss.[6] Several familial syndromes increase the risk of having a meningioma up to 50% (Box 1).[7]

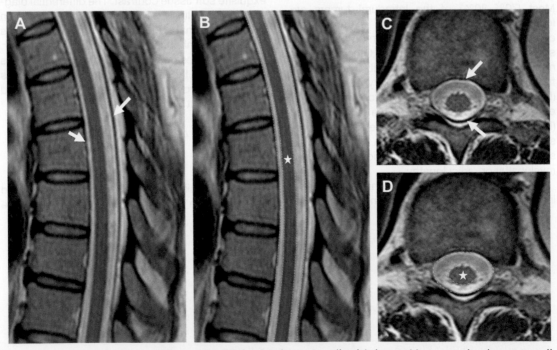

Fig. 1. The intradural extramedullary space (highlighted area in yellow) is located between the dura externally (*arrows* in A, C) and the surface of the cord (*star* in B, D) internally.

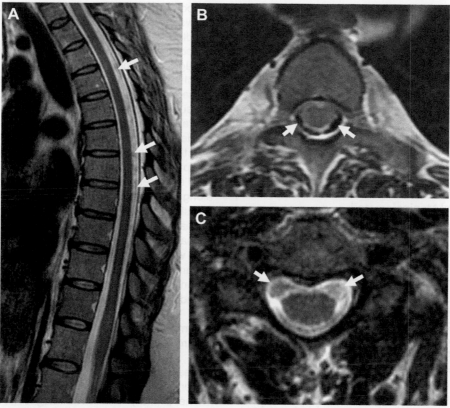

Fig. 2. CSF flow-related artifacts. T2WI MR imaging of the spine in three different patients (*A–C*) showing areas of low T2 signal within the intradural extramedullary space (*arrows*) resulting from turbulence and artifacts associated with CSF flow.

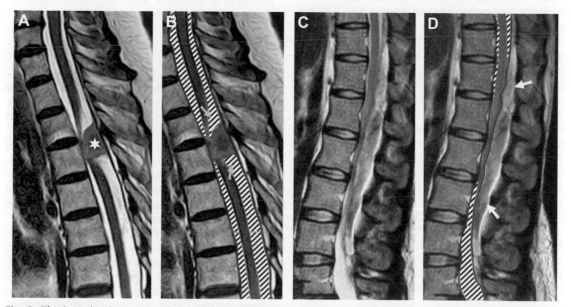

Fig. 3. The intradural versus epidural space. Sagittal T2WI images of the spine. The dura is outlined in red, and the intradural extramedullary space with diagonal stripes in *B* and *D*. Patient 1 (*A, B*) has a lesion (*star* in *A*) in the intradural extramedullary space. The lesion compresses the cord, enlarging the subarachnoid space at the tumor margins (*arrows* in *B*). Patient 2 (*C, D*) has a hematoma in the posterior epidural space (*arrows* in *D*), with resultant narrowing of the intradural space.

Spinal meningiomas occur most commonly in middle-aged women with a female/male ratio of 4–5:1.[8] Approximately, 80% are located in the thoracic spine, 15% in the cervical spine, and 5% in the lumbar spine. The intradural space is the most common site of involvement in 90% of spinal meningiomas.[4] Patients usually present with gait ataxia, radicular pain, and motor and sensory deficits due to chronic compressive myelopathy or radiculopathy.[5,8]

On MR imaging, intradural meningiomas are typically well-circumscribed lesions with a broad dural base, isointense to hypointense on T1WI and slightly hyperintense on T2WI relative to the spinal cord. Intense solid enhancement on post-contrast images is typical. The "dural tail" sign is seen in up to 70% of cases (Fig. 4).[9] Punctate or coarse calcifications might be present on CT, and hyperostosis is rare. The "ginkgo leaf sign" is highly specific for a meningioma arising lateral or ventrolateral to the spinal cord.[10] The name of this sign derives from a fan-shaped spinal cord and a streak within the tumor (Fig. 5). The primary differential diagnosis of a spinal meningioma is a nerve sheath tumor.

Complete surgical resection is the treatment of choice. Risk factors associated with recurrence include younger age, foraminal location, and en plaque growth pattern.[11] Stereotactic radiation is considered in poor surgical candidates, incomplete resection, higher grade tumors, or local recurrence.

Schwannoma

Spinal schwannoma accounts for 15% to 50% of intradural extramedullary spinal masses.[5] This is a WHO grade 1 tumor arising from the nerves' supporting Schwann cells. On histopathology, schwannomas show a biphasic pattern of cellular bundles (Antoni A) and a less cellular cobweb-like component (Antoni B). Cystic changes or hemorrhage are common in large lesions.[12]

Schwannoma tumorigenesis involves the loss of merlin expression, the growth inhibitory protein of neurofibromatosis type 2 (NF2), in up to 75% of sporadic tumors.[13] Schwannomas have a peak incidence at 40 to 50 years of age, without sex predilection. Clinical manifestations include sensory symptoms or symptoms related to nerve root or cord compression, given the more common origin along the dorsal intradural space. Schwannomas are slow-growing lesions with an annual volume increase of 2% to 7%.[14,15]

Imaging appearance varies depending on histology, with a heterogeneous MR imaging signal and enhancement seen in tumors with predominant Antoni B components. Classic MR imaging features include a well-circumscribed, T1WI iso-hypointense and T2WI hyperintense enhancing mass, more commonly arising from the dorsal nerve roots. Internal areas of cystic degeneration are commonly seen (Fig. 6). Large lesions can show a heterogeneous appearance secondary to hemorrhage or cystic degeneration and can mimic MPE (Fig. 7).

The primary differential diagnosis is neurofibroma when the tumor is solitary and drop metastases in cases of multiple small schwannomas. Schwannomas do not usually recur if gross total resection is achieved, and malignant transformation is exceptionally rare.[16]

Neurofibromatosis Type 2 and Schwannomatosis

NF2 is an autosomal dominant disease caused by a pathological sequence variant of the *NF2* gene, characterized by multiple benign tumors and dysplastic/hamartomatous lesions in the CNS, including multiple schwannomas (mainly bilateral vestibular schwannomas), meningiomas, and spinal ependymomas. It affects 2.5 to 4 per 100 000 individuals with no racial or sex preference.[17] About half of NF2 cases are sporadic, and greater than 50% of de novo cases are somatic mosaics.[18]

NF2-associated schwannomas differ from sporadic tumors as they occur in younger patients (30 vs 60 years). In addition to having larger schwannomas, patients with NF2 may have numerous small Schwann cell tumorlets on peripheral nerves and spinal nerves (Fig. 8).[19] Hybrid schwannoma–neurofibroma lesions are common in NF2, accounting for 30% of NF2 schwannomas.[20]

Schwannomatosis (SWN) is characterized by multiple schwannomas and less commonly

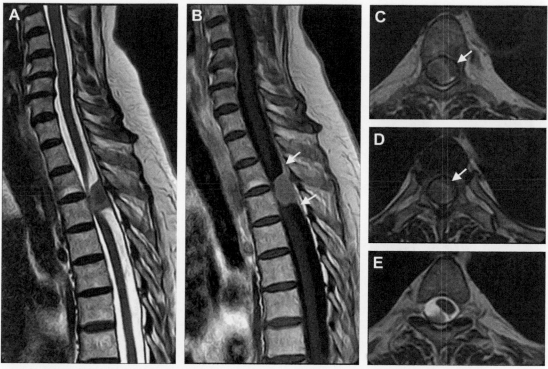

Fig. 4. Meningioma. A dural-based lesion in the posterior intradural extramedullary space shows low T2 signal (*A* and *E*) and avid enhancement (*B*). A dural tail can be seen in the sagittal T1WI post-gadolinium image (*arrows* in *B*). The lesion compresses the cord (*arrows* in *C, D*), which is flattened and anteriorly displaced.

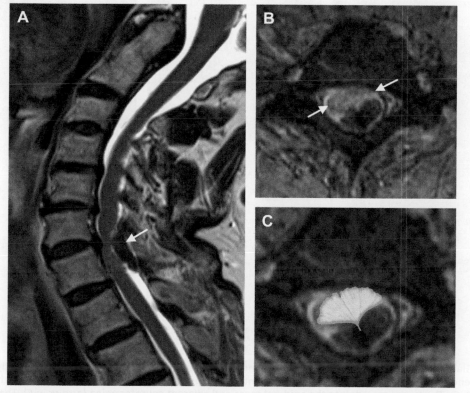

Fig. 5. Ginkgo leaf sign. Sagittal T2WI MR imaging (*A*) shows a posterior intradural meningioma of low signal (*arrow* in *A*) in the lower cervical canal. Axial T2WI (*B*) demonstrates the anterior displacement and compression of the cord (*arrows in B*), which acquires a characteristic "ginkgo leaf" configuration (*C*).

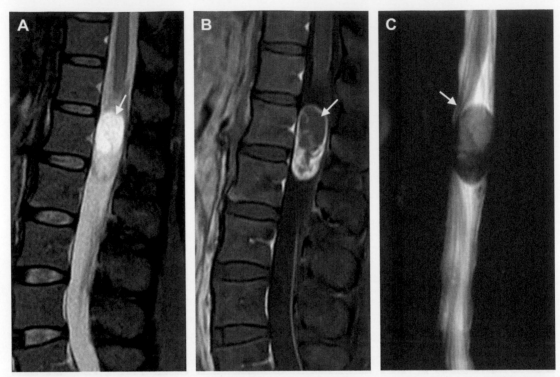

Fig. 6. Intradural extramedullary schwannoma with cystic degeneration. The lesion shows a high T2 signal (*arrow* in *A*) and a nonenhancing (*arrow* in *B*) cystic tumor component. The mass displaces the conus medullaris and proximal roots of the cauda equina (*arrow* in *C*).

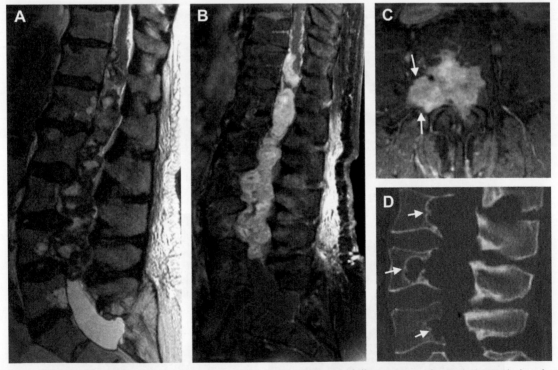

Fig. 7. Giant schwannoma. Large heterogeneous intradural extramedullary mass with predominantly low but heterogenous T2WI signal (*A*) and avid enhancement on the sagittal and axial post-contrast T1WI with fat saturation (*B, C*). The tumor extends into the epidural space and adjacent neuroforamina (*arrows* in *C*). There is associated smooth scalloping of the posterior wall of several vertebral bodies on CT (*arrows* in *D*), indicative of a slowly growing mass.

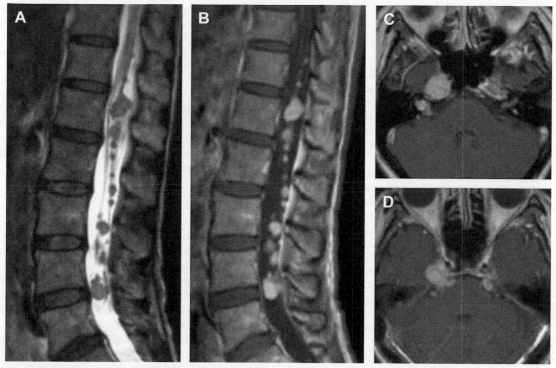

Fig. 8. Neurofibromatosis 2. Multiple intradural nodules of low T2 signal (*A*) and homogeneous enhancement on post-contrast T1WI (*B*) within the cauda equina. Associated bilateral vestibular and trigeminal schwannomas (*C, D*).

meningiomas in young adults without germline NF2 mutations. Fifteen percent of patients have a positive family history with autosomal dominant transmission but incomplete penetrance.[21] Genes implicated in SWN include SMARCB1 and LZTR1, both located on chromosome 22. Germline mutations in these genes account for 70% to 80% of familial SWN. Around 30% of SWN cases are sporadic.[22]

Importantly, 37% to 57% of patients fulfilling sporadic SWN criteria with no SMARCB1 and LZTR1 germline mutations end up having a mosaic NF2.[22] As the phenotype of these diseases spans a continuum with significant overlapping features,[23] a new classification proposal suggests using the umbrella term SWN along with the gene affected (Table 1).

Patients with SWN typically have multiple schwannomas in the spinal nerve roots and less commonly cranial nerves (Fig. 9). Most lesions (~70%) are hybrid schwannoma neurofibroma tumors with prominent myxoid stroma.[20,24] Severe tumor-associated chronic pain is characteristic, whereas neurologic deficits and polyneuropathy are uncommon.[24] Life expectancy in SWN is near normal and even higher than in patients with NF2.[25]

Neurofibroma

Neurofibroma is a benign peripheral nerve sheath tumor. It consists of mature neoplastic Schwann cells intermixed with nonneoplastic cell types. Unlike schwannomas, they lack Antoni A cell population and typically have normal peripheral nerve fibers intermixed within the tumor. All histologic subtypes are considered WHO grade 1, except for atypical neurofibromatous neoplasm of uncertain biological potential, which has no assigned tumor grade.[26]

Tumorigenesis of neurofibromas involves a biallelic genetic inactivation of the neurofibromatosis type 1 (*NF1*) gene in a Schwann cell subpopulation.[27] Neurofibroma most commonly affects the skin, with medium-sized nerves, nerve plexus, or a major nerve trunk less commonly involved. Spinal neurofibromas are typically located in the cervical region. Bilateral involvement of multiple spinal roots is typical of NF1. Cranial nerve involvement is exceptional. Most patients with a neurofibroma are asymptomatic. Larger tumors may cause motor and sensory deficits.

Spinal neurofibromas can have different macroscopic appearances: focal, diffuse, or plexiform morphology. Therefore, the imaging characteristics can range from a small, well-defined lesion along the course of a spinal nerve to large transpatial masses along various peripheral nerves. Neurofibromas typically show a marked T2WI/short tau inversion recovery (STIR) hyperintensity, which can help differentiate them from a schwannoma

Table 1
Proposed nomenclature for multiple schwannomas

Proposed Term	Definition
NF2-related schwannomatosis	Multiple schwannomas in the context of NF2
SMARCB1-related Schwannomatosis LZTR1-related S chwannomatosis	Multiple schwannomas in the context of Schwannomatosis
22-q related Schwannomatosis	Multiple schwannomas with common molecular findings on chromosome 22q
Schwannomatosis-not otherwise specified	Clinical features of NF2 or schwannomatosis, but without a molecular analysis
Schwannomatosis-not elsewhere classified	Molecular analysis of blood and tumors has failed to detect a genetic mutation.

Data from Plotkin SR, Messiaen L, Legius E, et al. Updated diagnostic criteria and nomenclature for neurofibromatosis type 2 and schwannomatosis: An international consensus recommendation. Genet Med. 2022;24(9):1967-1977.

and intense enhancement after contrast administration (Fig. 10). Larger lesions may have heterogenous signal and enhancement due to cystic degeneration and hemorrhage. The "target sign" (central T2 hyperintensity with peripheral T2 hypointensity) is suggestive but not specific for a neurofibroma (see Fig. 10). As with schwannomas, intradural and extramedullary neurofibromas extend through a widened neuroforamen. Plexiform neurofibromas are seen as large soft tissue masses with a "bag of worms" appearance.[12,28]

Because neurofibromas lack a capsule and some normal peripheral nerves are intermixed within the tumor, complete resection with nerve preservation is impossible. Close observation is currently the treatment of choice.

Myxopapillary Ependymoma

Spinal MPE is a slow-growing WHO grade 2 variant of spinal cord ependymoma originating from filum terminale glial cells. MPE is the most prevalent primary neoplasm of the conus medullaris and cauda equina. It has a male predominance (2:1) and predilection for young adults, with a mean age of 36 years at presentation. Up to 8% to 20% MPEs are found in pediatric patients.[29]

Patients present clinically with subacute or chronic low back pain, weakness, numbness in the lower extremities, saddle hypoesthesia, and sexual dysfunction.[30] MPEs are encapsulated masses showing mucinous and papillary zones intermixed with cellular rosettes and pseudorosettes on histopathology.[31]

On imaging, MPE appears as an avidly enhancing intradural extramedullary sausage-shaped mass in the cauda equina, abutting the

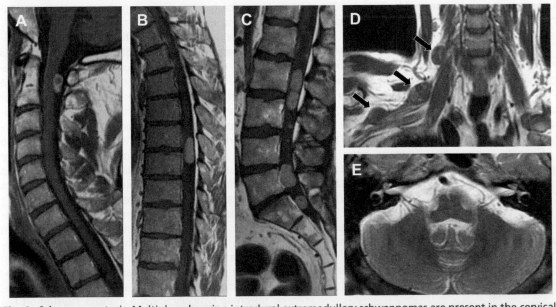

Fig. 9. Schwannomatosis. Multiple enhancing intradural extramedullary schwannomas are present in the cervical, thoracic, and lumbosacral spine (*A–C*). Additional schwannomas are present in the right brachial plexus (*arrows* in *D*). Note the absence of vestibular schwannomas within the internal auditory canals and cerebellopontine angles (*E*).

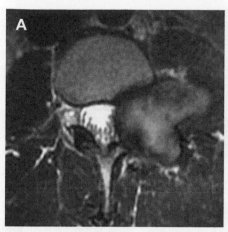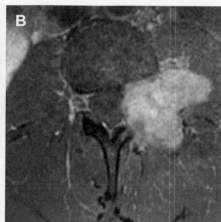

Fig. 10. Neurofibroma. There is a solid intradural-extradural mass within a left lumbar neuroforamen showing central T2 hyperintensity (*A*) with peripheral T2 hypointensity ("target sign") and avid enhancement on post-contrast T1 (*B*).

conus (Fig. 11). Larger lesions may expand the spinal canal and extend into the neuroforamina. MR imaging demonstrates isointense signal on T1WI and high signal on T2WI compared with the spinal cord. A heterogeneous signal can be found due to mucus or blood products.

Slow unremitting bleeding may result in a linear magnetic susceptibility artifact along the lesion margins, known as the "cap sign," reflecting hemosiderin deposition. Avid enhancement is the norm in post-contrast imaging.[4] The determination of conus involvement is critical in the preoperative imaging assessment, given that when present, gross total resection becomes difficult and carries a higher risk of tumor capsule rupture (Fig. 12).[32] Although MPE usually presents as a solitary lesion; efforts should be made to document multifocal disease. CSF dissemination or "drop metastases" is a known but uncommon phenomenon (Fig. 13).[33]

Gross total resection offers the best outcomes in terms of lower recurrence rate and risk of metastasis compared with subtotal resection. Disease recurrence may be seen in up to 40% of patients undergoing subtotal resection and up to 15% following gross total resection. Recurrence is linked to tumor capsule violation during surgical removal. In cases of subtotal resection or capsular violation, adjuvant focal radiotherapy improves progression-free survival (PFS). Craniospinal radiation is recommended for patients with documented cranial or spinal metastatic disease on imaging or CSF.[34] Drop metastases at presentation increase the likelihood of recurrence even when the postoperative imaging is negative for residual disease.[35]

Despite the high rate of recurrence and metastasis, 90% of patients have favorable outcomes following treatment. The 10-year overall survival rate is 92%, and the 10-year PFS is ~61%.[36]

MALIGNANT TUMORS
Leptomeningeal Metastasis

Leptomeningeal metastasis (LM) is frequently seen in the setting of advanced cancer. It occurs in 5% to 8% of patients with solid tumors and in 5% to 15% of hematologic malignancies.[37] Lower motor weakness, radicular signs, sensory changes, ataxia, and bowel or bladder dysfunction in a patient with cancer should alert for LM.[38] The average survival of patients with LM is 2 to 4 months despite treatment.[37]

To establish a definitive diagnosis, neoplastic cells should be found in CSF cytology. However, in some instances, this could remain negative. The positivity rate of CSF cytology increases after multiple lumbar punctures, from approximately 50% after a single sample to 85% to 90% following three repeated lumbar taps.[39]

In the proper clinical scenario, post-contrast MR imaging is accurate to establish the diagnosis of LM, even when CSF cytology is inconclusive. Abnormal nodular enhancement, predominantly in the cauda equina, supports the diagnosis (Fig. 14). A curvilinear enhancement in the topography of intrathecal nerve roots is suggestive but less specific. When these imaging findings are evaluated in conjunction with the clinical context, MR imaging has a sensitivity of 70% and specificity of 77% to 100% for diagnosis confirmation.[39]

Lymphoma

While rare, lymphoma may affect the different compartments of the spine in the following frequency: bone, epidural space, intradural extramedullary space, and spinal cord.

Leptomeningeal lymphoma results from hematogenous dissemination, CSF spread, or perineural

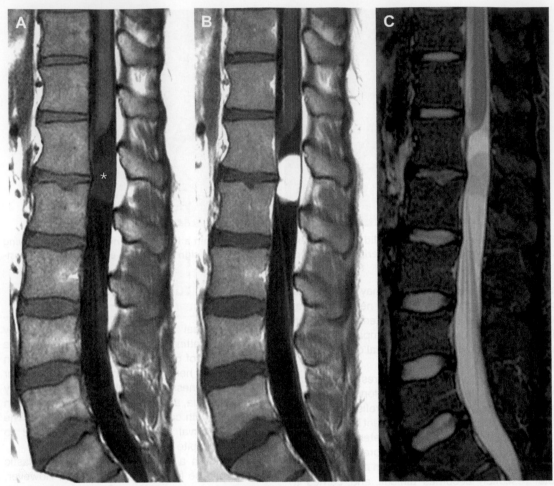

Fig. 11. There is an intradural mass along the proximal cauda equina (*asterisk* in *A*), showing low signal in the sagittal T1WI (*A*), avid homogeneous enhancement on post-contrast T1WI (*B*), and a high signal in the sagittal T2WI (*C*) consistent with a myxopapillary ependymoma.

extension of systemic lymphoma to the intradural extramedullary compartment. Post-gadolinium MR imaging reveals enhancing nodular lesions along the surface of the cord or nerve root thickening (Fig. 15). Diffusion weigthed imaging (DWI) may show non-facilitated diffusion due to increased cellularity.[40]

Malignant Peripheral Nerve Sheath Tumor

MPNST corresponds to less than 1% of all peripheral nerve neoplasms.[4] It is more common in adults with a mean age at presentation of 40 to 44 years.[4] Half of the cases occur in NF1, usually in young patients, arising from a preexisting neurofibroma or plexiform neurofibroma.[4] Forty percent are sporadic without a tumor precursor, and 10% develop after radiation therapy.

On imaging, features that suggest MPNST include an ill-defined margin, perilesional edema, intratumoral cystic degeneration, and heterogeneous enhancement (Fig. 16).[41] Malignant degeneration of a benign nerve sheath tumor should be suspected in lesions with nodular growing components, an isolated portion exhibiting disproportionate growth, and continued tumor growth during adulthood.

The standard treatment consists of surgical resection and adjuvant radiotherapy. Large size, high grade on histopathological analysis, prior radiation, and history of NF1 are poor prognostic factors.

OTHER RARE TUMORS
Solitary Fibrous Tumor

SFTs are connective tissue neoplasms composed of spindle cells on a background of collagen stroma.[42] Positiveness for signal transducer and activator of transcription 6 on nuclear immunostaining is the hallmark of SFT.[43] These tumors

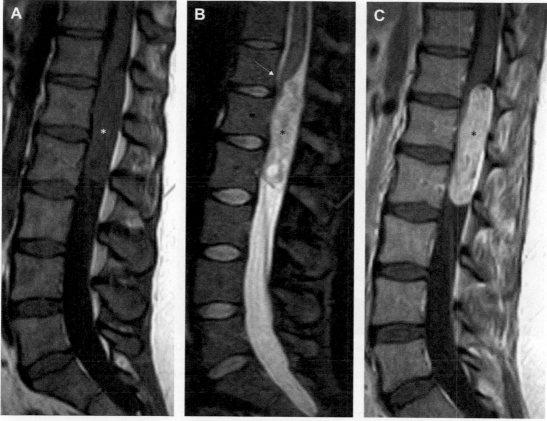

Fig. 12. Intradural extramedullary mass (*asterisk* in *A–C*) demonstrating heterogeneous signal intensity on sagittal T1WI (*A*) and T2WI (*B*), and avid enhancement on post-contrast T1WI (*C*). The proximal portion of the mass contacts the conus (*arrow* in *B*). At surgery, a myxopapillary ependymoma adherent to the conus was found.

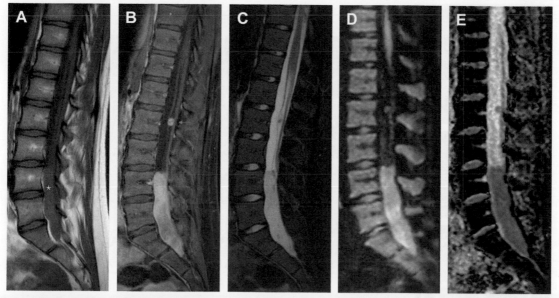

Fig. 13. Myxopapillary ependymoma with drop metastasis. A large intradural mass (*asterisk* in *A*) is present within the distal thecal sac, showing homogeneous post-contrast T1WI enhancement (*B*), high T2WI signal (*C*), and restricted diffusion (*D, E*). The mass creates mild scalloping of the posterior surface of L4 and L5 vertebral bodies. An additional 6-mm enhancing drop metastasis is present at the L2 level (*arrow* in *B*).

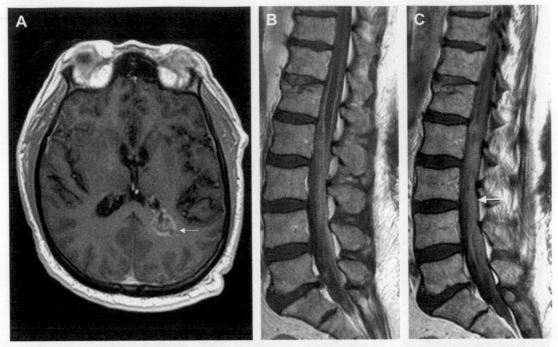

Fig. 14. Patient with periventricular IDH (−) glioblastoma (*white arrow* in A), and neurologic deficits in the lower extremities. Sagittal post-contrast T1WIs of the lumbar spine (*B* and *C*) show abnormal thickening and enhancement of the cauda equina nerve roots and multiple nodular enhancing lesions (*arrow* in *C*). CSF cytology confirmed leptomeningeal metastases. IDH, isocitrate dehydrogenase.

commonly occur in the pleura, with less than 2% presenting in the spine. Spinal pain is seen in about two-third of patients, followed by symptoms related to cord or radicular compression.[43]

The thoracic spine is the most common site of involvement in half of the patients, followed by the cervical and lumbar spine.[43] Within the spinal canal, up to 65% of SFT are intradural

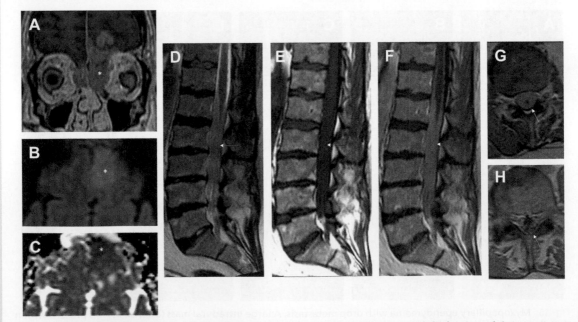

Fig. 15. Ethmoid lymphoma with intracranial extension (*asterisk* in A–C). Abnormal thickening of the nerve roots of the cauda equina on sagittal T2WI (*D*) and T1WI (*E*) (*arrows*), with associated diffuse enhancement on post-contrast T1 (*arrows* in *F–H*).

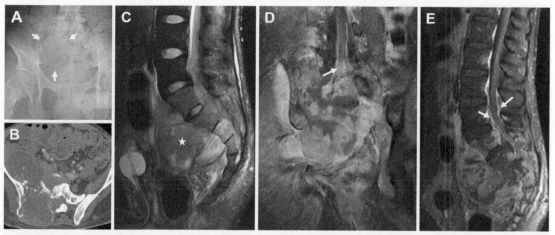

Fig. 16. Malignant peripheral nerve sheath tumor (MPSNT) in the context of NF1. Plain film of the pelvis shows an ill-defined lucency involving the right sacrum (*arrows in A*). Enhanced axial CT (*B*) demonstrates a large destructive mass centered in the right sacrum, ipsilateral presacral space, and posterior paraspinal soft tissues. The lesion is heterogenous with areas of low T2 signal reflecting high tumor cellularity (*star in C*). There is heterogenous enhancement on post-contrast T1WI (*D–E*) and tumor invasion of the intradural (*arrow in D*) and epidural spaces (*arrows in E*).

extramedullary in location, 26% are intradural and extradural, and 9% extradural.[43] On imaging, SFTs are usually isointense on T1WI and variable on T2WI (**Fig. 17**).[42] All tumors are associated with marked homogeneous or heterogeneous post-contrast enhancement. Calcification or hemorrhage is not seen. The presence of intralesional flow voids is uncommon. A complete surgical

removal is the first step toward diagnosis and treatment, but this is achieved in about two-thirds of patients due to bleeding or spinal cord invasion.[43]

Paraganglioma

Spinal paragangliomas are uncommon intradural extramedullary tumors. They usually occur in the

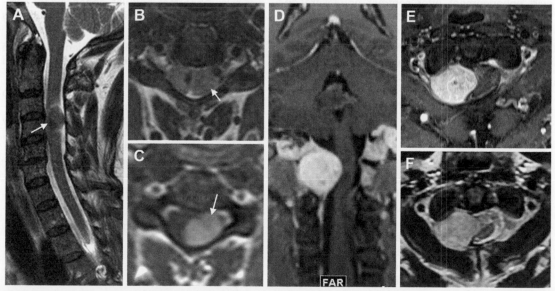

Fig. 17. Solitary fibrous tumors (SFT) in two patients. Patient 1 (*A–C*) has an intradural mass in the cervical spine of low T2WI signal (*arrow in A, B*) and avid post-contrast T1WI enhancement (*arrow in C*), causing significant mass effect on the cord. Patient 2 (*D–F*) has an intradural–extradural SFT in the upper cervical canal showing avid post-contrast enhancement (*D, E*) and nonhomogeneous T2WI signal (*F*).

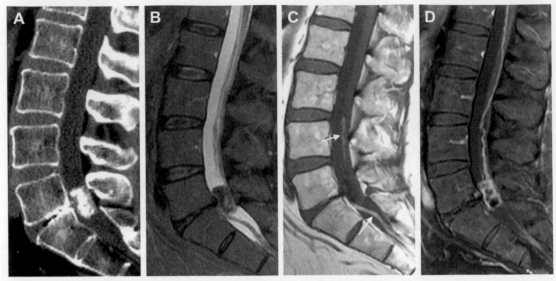

Fig. 18. Paraganglioma. Intradural lesion within the distal thecal sac showing the presence of calcifications (A) on CT, and low T2WI signal on MR imaging (B). Linear areas of high signal surrounding the mass on T1WI are suggestive of subacute hemorrhage (arrows in C). The lesion shows avid heterogeneous enhancement and a prominent vessel on T1WI post-contrast (D).

cauda equina, representing 4% of all tumors in this region.[4] The age at presentation ranges from 9 to 74 years, and males are more commonly affected. Back pain and sciatica are the most common symptoms.[4]

On imaging, spinal paraganglioma appears as a well-defined encapsulated mass with iso or hypointense signal on T1WI, high signal on T2WI, and avid enhancement after contrast administration (Fig. 18). The areas of low T2WI could be present within the lesion or along the superior margin, known as the "cap sign," which represents hemosiderin deposition. Prominent flow voids and cystic components can also be seen.[44] Surgical resection is usually curative, whereas incompletely resected tumors can be treated with adjuvant radiotherapy.

SUMMARY

Patients with intradural extramedullary tumors usually present with gait ataxia, radicular pain, and motor and sensory deficits due to chronic compressive myelopathy or radiculopathy. Contrast-enhanced MR imaging is the imaging modality of choice for the detection and evaluation of intradural extramedullary spinal tumors. Radiologists should be familiar with the key imaging features of common and infrequent tumors found within this compartment of the spine to help narrow the differential diagnosis and guide treatment.

CLINICS CARE POINTS

- In the proper clinical context, post-contrast MR imaging is accurate to establish the diagnosis of leptomeningeal metastases, even when cerebrospinal fluid cytology is inconclusive. Abnormal nodular enhancement, predominantly in the cauda equina, supports the diagnosis.

- In general, symptomatic patients or those with a rapidly growing tumor are surgical candidates.

- Surgical resection is the ideal therapy to achieve long-term tumor control in symptomatic patients with intradural extramedullary neoplasms, given that, for the most part, these are histologically benign.

DISCLOSURE

The authors have nothing to disclose.

REFERENCES

1. Duong LM, McCarthy BJ, McLendon RE, et al. Descriptive epidemiology of malignant and nonmalignant primary spinal cord, spinal meninges, and cauda equina tumors, United States, 2004-2007. Cancer 2012;118(17):4220–7.

2. Sensenig EC. The early development of the meninges of the spinal cord in human embryos. Carnegie Inst Washingt Contrib to Embryol 1951; 228(1816):145–57. v. 34. Available at: https://eurekamag.com/research/025/735/025735895.php. Accessed 27 November, 2022.

3. Lisanti C, Carlin C, Banks KP, et al. Normal MRI appearance and motion-related phenomena of CSF. Am J Roentgenol 2007;188(3):716–25.

4. Koeller KK, Shih RY. Intradural extramedullary spinal neoplasms: radiologic-pathologic correlation. Radiographics 2019;39(2):468–90.

5. Weber C, Gulati S, Jakola AS, et al. Incidence rates and surgery of primary intraspinal tumors in the era of modern neuroimaging: A national population-based study. Spine 2014;39(16). https://doi.org/10.1097/BRS.0000000000000412.

6. Torp SH, Solheim O, Skjulsvik AJ. The WHO 2021 Classification of Central Nervous System tumours: a practical update on what neurosurgeons need to know—a minireview. Acta Neurochir 2022;164(9): 2453–64.

7. Kerr K, Qualmann K, Esquenazi Y, et al. Familial syndromes involving meningiomas provide mechanistic insight into sporadic disease. Clin Neurosurg 2018; 83(6):1107–18.

8. Kshettry VR, Hsieh JK, Ostrom QT, et al. Descriptive epidemiology of spinal meningiomas in the United States. Spine 2015;40(15):E886–9.

9. Alorainy IA. Dural tail sign in spinal meningiomas. Eur J Radiol 2006;60(3):387–91.

10. Yamaguchi S, Takeda M, Takahashi T, et al. Ginkgo leaf sign: a highly predictive imaging feature of spinal meningioma. J Neurosurg Spine 2015;23(5): 642–6.

11. Park BJ, Dougherty MC, Noeller J, et al. Spinal meningioma in adults: imaging characteristics, surgical outcomes, and risk factors for recurrence. World Neurosurg 2022;164:e852–60.

12. Ledbetter LN, Leever JD. Imaging of intraspinal tumors. Radiol Clin North Am 2019;57(2):341–57.

13. Oh JE, Ohta T, Satomi K, et al. Alterations in the NF2/LATS1/LATS2/YAP pathway in Schwannomas. J Neuropathol Exp Neurol 2015;74(10):952–9.

14. Sun I, Pamir MN. Non-syndromic spinal schwannomas: a novel classification. Front Neurol 2017; 8(JUL):318.

15. Lenzi J, Anichini G, Landi A, et al. Spinal nerves schwannomas: experience on 367 cases - historic overview on how clinical, radiological, and surgical practices have changed over a course of 60 years. Neurol Res Int 2017;2017. https://doi.org/10.1155/2017/3568359.

16. McMenamin ME, Fletcher CDM. Expanding the spectrum of malignant change in schwannomas: Epithelioid malignant change, epithelioid malignant peripheral nerve sheath tumor, and epithelioid angiosarcoma: a study of 17 cases. Am J Surg Pathol 2001;25(1):13–25.

17. Evans DGR, Moran A, King A, et al. Incidence of vestibular schwannoma and neurofibromatosis 2 in the North West of England over a 10-year period: Higher incidence than previously thought. Otol Neurotol 2005;26(1):93–7.

18. Evans DG, Hartley CL, Smith PT, et al. Incidence of mosaicism in 1055 de novo NF2 cases: much higher than previous estimates with high utility of next-generation sequencing. Genet Med 2020;22(1): 53–9.

19. Stemmer-Rachamimov AO, Ino Y, Lim ZY, et al. Loss of the NF2 gene and merlin occur by the tumorlet stage of schwannoma development in neurofibromatosis 2. J Neuropathol Exp Neurol 1998;57(12): 1164–7.

20. Harder A, Wesemann M, Hagel C, et al. Hybrid neurofibroma/schwannoma is overrepresented among schwannomatosis and neurofibromatosis patients. Am J Surg Pathol 2012;36(5):702–9.

21. MacCollin M, Willett C, Heinrich B, et al. Familial schwannomatosis: Exclusion of the NF2 locus as the germline event. Neurology 2003;60(12):1968–74.

22. Plotkin SR, Messiaen L, Legius E, et al. Updated diagnostic criteria and nomenclature for neurofibromatosis type 2 and schwannomatosis: An international consensus recommendation. Genet Med 2022;24(9):1967–77.

23. Smith MJ, Isidor B, Beetz C, et al. Mutations in LZTR1 add to the complex heterogeneity of schwannomatosis. Neurology 2015;84(2):141–7.

24. Merker VL, Esparza S, Smith MJ, et al. Clinical features of schwannomatosis: a retrospective analysis of 87 patients. Oncol 2012;17(10):1317–22.

25. Evans DG, Bowers NL, Tobi S, et al. Schwannomatosis: a genetic and epidemiological study. J Neurol Neurosurg Psychiatr 2018;89(11):1215–9.

26. Louis DN, Perry A, Wesseling P, et al. The 2021 WHO classification of tumors of the central nervous system: a summary. Neuro Oncol 2021;23(8): 1231–51.

27. Liao CP, Booker RC, Brosseau JP, et al. Contributions of inflammation and tumor microenvironment to neurofibroma tumorigenesis. J Clin Invest 2018; 128(7):2848–61.

28. Soldatos T, Fisher S, Karri S, et al. Advanced MR imaging of peripheral nerve sheath tumors including diffusion imaging. Semin Musculoskelet Radiol 2015;19(2):179–90.

29. Sonneland PRL, Scheithauer BW, Onofrio BM. Myxopapillary ependymoma. A clinicopathologic and immunocytochemical study of 77 cases. Cancer 1985;56(4):883–93.

30. Liu T, Yang C, Deng X, et al. Clinical characteristics and surgical outcomes of spinal myxopapillary ependymomas. Neurosurg Rev 2020;43(5):1351–6.

31. Koeller KK, Rosenblum RS, Morrison AL. From the archives of the AFIP neoplasms of the spinal cord and filum terminale: Radiologie-pathologie correlation. Radiographics 2000;20(6):1721–49.

32. Al-Habib A, Al-Radi OO, Shannon P, et al. Myxopapillary ependymoma: correlation of clinical and imaging features with surgical resectability in a series with long-term follow-up. Spinal Cord 2011;49(10):1073–8.

33. Kraetzig T, McLaughlin L, Bilsky MH, et al. Metastases of spinal myxopapillary ependymoma: Unique characteristics and clinical management. J Neurosurg Spine 2018;28(2):201–8.

34. Chao ST, Kobayashi T, Benzel E, et al. The role of adjuvant radiation therapy in the treatment of spinal myxopapillary ependymomas: clinical article. J Neurosurg Spine 2011;14(1):59–64.

35. Tabor JK, Ryu B, Schneider D, et al. Multifocal lumbar myxopapillary ependymoma presenting with drop metastasis: a case report and review of the literature. Spinal Cord Ser Cases 2022;8(1). https://doi.org/10.1038/s41394-022-00513-x.

36. Weber DC, Wang Y, Miller R, et al. Long-term outcome of patients with spinal myxopapillary ependymoma: treatment results from the MD Anderson Cancer Center and institutions from the Rare Cancer Network. Neuro Oncol 2014;17(4):588–95.

37. Wang N, Bertalan MS, Brastianos PK. Leptomeningeal metastasis from systemic cancer: review and update on management. Cancer 2018;124(1):21–35.

38. DeAngelis LM. Current diagnosis and treatment of leptomeningeal metastasis. J Neuro Oncol 1998;38:245–52.

39. Freilich RJ, Krol G, Deangelis LM. Neuroimaging and cerebrospinal fluid cytology in the diagnosis of leptomeningeal metastasis. Ann Neurol 1995;38(1):51–7.

40. Haque S, Law M, Abrey LE, et al. Imaging of lymphoma of the central nervous system, spine, and orbit. Radiol Clin North Am 2008;46(2):339–61.

41. Wilson MP, Katlariwala P, Low G, et al. Diagnostic accuracy of MRI for the detection of malignant peripheral nerve sheath tumors: a systematic review and meta-analysis. Am J Roentgenol 2021;217(1):31–9.

42. Ginat DT, Bokhari A, Bhatt S, et al. Imaging features of solitary fibrous tumors. Am J Roentgenol 2011;196(3):487–95.

43. Apra C, Arbi A El, Montero AS, et al. Spinal solitary fibrous tumors: an original multicenter series and systematic review of presentation, management, and prognosis. Cancers 2022;14(12). https://doi.org/10.3390/cancers14122839.

44. Merhemic Z, Stosic-Opincal T, Thurnher MM. Neuroimaging of Spinal Tumors. Magn Reson Imaging Clin N Am 2016;24(3):563–79.

Troublemaking Lesions
Spinal Tumor Mimics

Kassie McCullagh, MD*, Carlos Zamora, MD, PhD, Mauricio Castillo, MD

KEYWORDS

- Spine • Tumor • Neoplasia • Mimic

KEY POINTS

- There are several mass-like lesions that can mimic true neoplasms in the spine, including vascular, inflammatory, infectious, congenital, and degenerative etiologies.
- Some spinal lesions have distinguishing imaging features on the basis of their morphology, location, extent, and other MR imaging findings such as the pattern of enhancement or presence of restricted diffusion.
- Several entities have overlapping imaging features and their diagnosis requires knowledge of the patient's history, clinical presentation, epidemiology, and/or laboratory findings.

INTRODUCTION

In the evaluation of spinal tumor-like lesions, consideration of potential mimics is important to avoid unnecessary biopsy, surgery, and treatments. Here, we review important spinal tumor mimics and discuss helpful imaging features to avoid mistaking these lesions for true neoplasias. While a precise diagnosis is not always possible by imaging, as many lesions have overlapping features, we review some of the characteristics that strongly support benign entities and influence patient management.

DISCUSSION

Dividing intradural lesions into intramedullary versus extramedullary is helpful when facing spinal cord lesions. Non-neoplastic intramedullary lesions have broad etiologies with major categories including vascular, inflammatory, and infectious causes while extramedullary lesions are often cysts related to an abnormal development, but can also be acquired. Some extradural lesions that can mimic masses and cause neurological symptoms are highlighted in this review.

Intramedullary Lesions

The majority of mass-like lesions of the cord are neoplastic, but when clinical and imaging findings do not suggest tumors, the differential diagnosis should include non-neoplastic processes as per later in discussion.

Vascular lesions

Cavernous malformations (CM) are not neoplastic and the term "cavernoma" is a misnomer. CM are comprised of multiple abnormal vascular channels lined by endothelial cells and are considered low-flow vascular malformations.[1] They are more common in the brain with less well-known epidemiology in the cord, with spinal CM comprising approximately 5% of intramedullary lesions in adults and 1% in the pediatric population.[2,3] Most cases of cerebral CM are sporadic (approximately 80%), but there are familial cerebral CM syndromes that predispose patients to spinal CM.[4]

Typical features of spinal CM are similar to cerebral CM including a well-demarcated lesion with a heterogenous signal on T1 and T2 weighted images due to the presence of blood

Division of Neuroradiology, Department of Radiology, The University of North Carolina, CB 7510 2000 Old Clinic, 101 Manning Drive, Chapel Hill, NC 27599, USA
* Corresponding author.
E-mail address: kassie_mccullagh@med.unc.edu

Neuroimag Clin N Am 33 (2023) 423–441
https://doi.org/10.1016/j.nic.2023.03.003
1052-5149/23/© 2023 Elsevier Inc. All rights reserved.

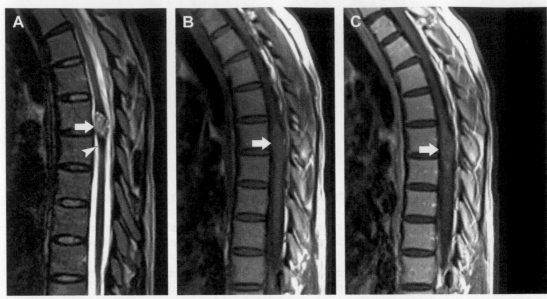

Fig. 1. Spinal cord cavernous malformation. Sagittal T2WI (*A*) shows a typical "popcorn" appearance (*arrow*) of a cavernous malformation with peripheral deposition of hemosiderin (*arrowhead*). Sagittal pre- (*B*) and post-contrast (*C*) T1WI show a few subtle foci of contrast enhancement. The appearance of CM is typical and easily distinguishable from tumors.

products of various ages resulting in the typical "popcorn appearance" (Fig. 1).[5] Due to peripheral hemosiderin deposition, a T2 hypointense rim is common with blooming on T2* GRE sequences.[5,6] Contrast enhancement is rare and generally minimal when present.[5] CM are most commonly seen in the thoracic cord[5,7] and can be intradural, extramedullary, or extradural.[8] Gradient-echo-based sequences are more sensitive for the detection of spinal CM as many lesions are small and may only be seen as small foci of hypointense signal.[4]

Occasionally spinal CM may bleed and result in frank hematomyelia. Tumors such as metastases may also bleed but often have extensive accompanying intramedullary edema. Ependymomas may also bleed but often present with internal chronic blood products and caps of hemosiderin/ferritin in their superior and inferior borders. Hemangioblastomas also occasionally bleed, but these hemorrhages tend to be acute and thus easily distinguishable from those of CM which are mostly chronic. Intramedullary arteriovenous malformations may present with hemorrhage and, in the absence of vascular nidus with flow voids, they may be extremely difficult to differentiate from CM and their diagnosis may necessitate catheter angiography.

Dural arteriovenous fistulas (dAVF) and arteriovenous malformations (AVM) are often extramedullary but discussed here, as associated edema may mimic a tumor. AVMs can sometimes be intramedullary. Key to their diagnosis is the recognition of serpentine vessels along the surface of the spinal cord that may be subtle on conventional MR imaging sequences (Fig. 2). These vessels are easier to detect with heavily T2-weighted high-resolution sequences such as SPACE, CISS, or FIESTA.

Spinal dAVF are associated with a long segment cord enlargement and edema commonly involving the lower thoracic cord and conus medullaris, although other sites of involvement are possible. Enhancement of the spinal cord is common and is due to venous congestion and in some cases, it can be intense (see Fig. 2). The levels of cord edema do not necessarily correlate with the fistula's location.[9] Spinal dAVF may be mistaken for a tumor, especially a glial infiltrative one, but these tumors generally do not show enlarged blood vessels (veins) on the spinal cord surface, except for myxopapillary ependymomas and paragangliomas. Another important finding is that edema caused by dAVF involves the central spinal cord, often leaving a rim of normal or slightly T2 hypointense signal along its periphery, a finding not present in tumors or demyelinating/inflammatory lesions where the entire transverse diameter of the cord tends to be involved.

Spinal AVMs are another type of vascular malformation encountered in the spine. The vascular

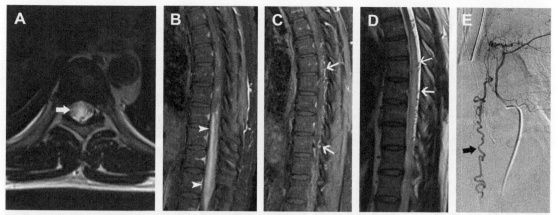

Fig. 2. Spinal dAVF. Axial T2WI (*A*) shows expansion and abnormal hyperintense signal of the spinal cord (*thick white arrow*). Sagittal post-contrast T1WI (*B*) shows extensive contrast enhancement involving the lower cord and extending to the conus medullaris (*arrowheads*). Sagittal post-contrast T1WI (*C*) and T2WI (*D*) show multiple prominent vessels along the dorsal surface of the cord, consistent with engorged draining veins (*thin arrows*). Frontal view digital subtraction angiography (*E*) confirms the dAVF with an engorged draining vein (*black arrow*) following injection of a thoracic radicular artery. Although the edema and contrast enhancement of the cord may suggest a tumor, the presence of large veins on the cord surface makes the diagnosis of dAVF almost certain.

nidus in AVMs can be located intramedullary or perimedullary, with some types also having paraspinal osseous or soft tissue components.[10] Altered vascular flow dynamics can lead to myelopathy from venous congestion, hemorrhage, and arterial steal from the cord.[11] Various classification systems exist for spinal vascular malformations and discussion of them is beyond the scope of this article, but care should be taken to specify the system used if reporting a specific type of AVM when interpreting MR imaging findings. As stated above, spinal AVM may mimic a CM, and distinguishing between them may be difficult.

Cord infarction *Anterior spinal artery syndrome* is most common and presents with bilateral paralysis below the affected level, and loss of pain and temperature sensation, with relative sparing of proprioception and vibration due to the sparing of the dorsal columns. On MR imaging, there is bilateral cord involvement due to a single anterior midline artery, with hyperintense signal on T2WI within the anterior and central cord (2/3s of the cord). Often the anterior horn cells have more pronounced signal changes which on axial imaging acutely will lead to the "owl eye appearance,"[12] formed by 2 small hyperintense dots in the anterior cord that span several levels. There can be a pronounced involvement including a larger central component of the cord, with only a thin rim of preserved surrounding peripheral white matter.[12] The adjacent vertebral bodies can also be infarcted and bone marrow signal changes can be a helpful diagnostic finding, however, this is seen

occasionally. DWI sequence can confirm ischemia within the cord (Fig. 3).[13–15] Although the clinical findings generally suggest this entity, by imaging it should be distinguished from rapidly progressing lymphoma which may also show restricted diffusion, abnormal T2 signal, and contrast enhancement. Distinction from inflammatory lesions, as described in the paragraph immediately below, is also important.

Posterior spinal artery syndrome is usually unilateral due to the involvement of one or both paired posterior spinal arteries. Clinical signs include complete sensory loss at the level of injury and loss of proprioception and vibration senses below the level. On imaging, hyperintense signal on T2WI is usually restricted to the paramedian dorsal columns.[13–15] The differential diagnosis includes other rare entities such as subacute combined degeneration, HIV-associated myelitis, syphilis, and decompression illness but the clinical presentation of these entities allows for the correct imaging diagnosis. Neoplasias tend to be shorter in length, present different patterns of contrast enhancement, and generally involve the entire transverse diameter of the cord and not only segments of it as do arterial infarctions. Demyelinating lesions may show segmental involvement but are shorter in length and tend to be restricted to the white matter tracts of the cord. Other inflammatory lesions such as acute disseminated encephalomyelitis (ADEM), neuromyelitis optica (NMO)-spectrum disorders, MOG myelitis, and idiopathic transverse myelitis (TM) also present acutely but are long lesions that tend to involve the entire

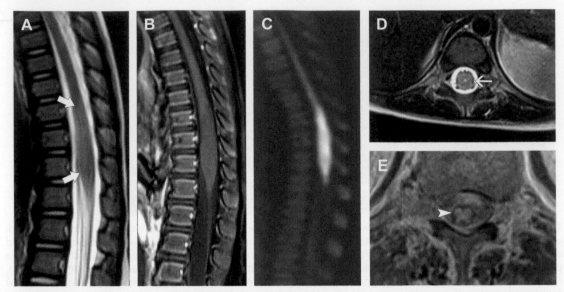

Fig. 3. Spinal cord infarction. Sagittal T2WI (*A*) and post-contrast T1WI (*B*) show the expansion of the distal cord and conus (*thick arrows* in *A*), without contrast enhancement. Note prominent restricted diffusion on DWI (*C*). Axial T2WI (*D*) shows entire involvement of the cross-sectional area of the cord (*thin arrow*). Axial T2WI in a different patient (*E*) shows a central pattern of signal abnormality, with preferential involvement of the anterior horns (*arrowhead*). Restricted diffusion may be seen with cord lymphoma but the acuteness of findings in cord infarctions should suggest the diagnosis as does the lack of enhancement and involvement of the gray matter shown in E.

transverse diameter of the cord. The acute clinical picture and serum markers help reach the correct imaging diagnosis.

Inflammation

A broad category of tumor mimics includes demyelination and inflammatory lesions. Cord edema and a tumefactive appearance of these lesions can make it difficult to distinguish actively demyelinating plaques from neoplasms. This issue is commonly encountered with multiple sclerosis (MS) but may also be seen with NMO-spectrum disorders, ADEM, and TM. Imaging of the brain, optic nerves, and CSF analysis are helpful in the diagnosis of these entities.

Multiple sclerosis

Cord abnormalities in MS follow a typical pattern of a short-segment signal abnormality, spanning less than 2 vertebral segments and with only partial involvement of the cross-sectional area of the cord.[16] On postcontrast imaging, their enhancement is variable, with rim or patchy enhancement (Fig. 4) seen in active lesions and no enhancement in chronic ones.[17] Of note, isolated cord lesions without intracranial lesions are seen in 10% to 20% of cases of MS.[17] Their imaging features are typical, and nearly always they can easily be distinguished from tumors.

Neuromyelitis optica spectrum disorders

NMO can have similar clinical features to MS, but its imaging findings can help distinguish between the 2 pathologies. Spinal cord involvement in NMO is usually longer (3 or more vertebral segments) and there is greater cross-sectional involvement of the cord than in MS.[18] Also, NMO lesions often show heterogenous hyperintense signal on T2WI, often described as "bright spotty lesions."[19] Presence of a long-segment cervical cord lesion extending to the area postrema is typical of NMO (Fig. 5). NMO is associated with optic neuritis which is more often bilateral and more severe than that seen in MS. Brain lesions in NMO are rare.[18] When in doubt, the imaging diagnosis is confirmed by the presence of positive aquaporin 4 IgG in serum.

Acute disseminated encephalomyelitis

ADEM is a monophasic condition more often seen in children with a prodrome of a viral infection.[20] ADEM can mimic MS, but usually has larger, ill-defined, and more mass-like lesions intracranially that can involve both white and gray matter, features which are less common in MS.[18] The cord lesions appear similar to TM with long segments of confluent hyperintense T2WI signal associated with cord expansion (Fig. 6).[18] Spinal cord involvement can present in isolation and is more

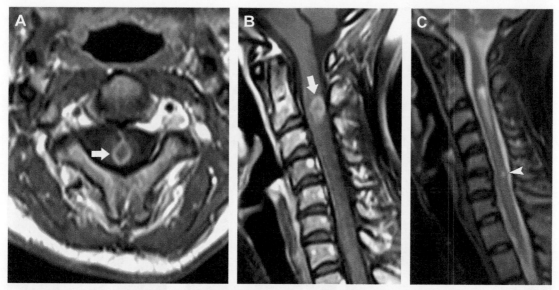

Fig. 4. Actively demyelinating plaque in multiple sclerosis. Axial (*A*) and sagittal (*B*) post-contrast T1WI show a peripherally enhancing lesion in the spinal cord at the C2-C3 level (*arrows*). Sagittal STIR (*C*) demonstrates the lesion with surrounding edema, as well as an additional smaller lesion at the C5-C6 level (*arrowhead*). Although the appearance of this plaque may be confused with tumor, the acuteness of symptoms, gender, younger age, and presence of MS lesions elsewhere generally aids in reaching the proper diagnosis.

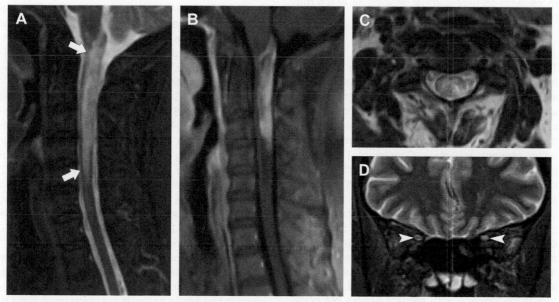

Fig. 5. Neuromyelitis optica. Sagittal STIR (*A*) shows longitudinally extensive and mildly expansile spinal cord signal abnormality extending to the area postrema (*arrows*). There is avid post-contrast enhancement (*B*). Axial T2WI (*C*) shows near total cross-sectional involvement of the cord with more discrete hyperintense foci consistent with "bright spotty lesions." Coronal T2WI (*D*) shows bilateral optic nerve atrophy with abnormal signal on the left (*arrowheads*) in keeping with sequelae of prior optic neuritis. Findings of NMOSD which help differentiate it from tumor include extension to the area postrema, involvement of the posterior optic nerves and chiasm, and positive antibodies (IgG) against aquaporin-4.

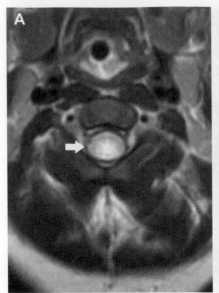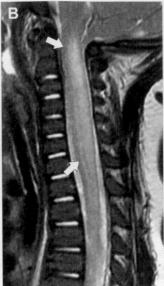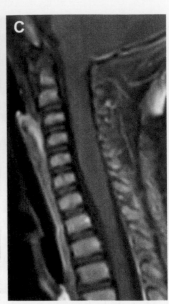

Fig. 6. ADEM. Axial (*A*) and sagittal (*B*) T2WI show extensive edema involving the entire cervical cord which has an expansile appearance (*arrows*). There is no associated contrast enhancement (*C*). Differentiating these lesions from an infiltrative glioma or glioneuronal tumor may be difficult, but ADEM usually has an acute presentation and responds to steroids, immune globulin, or plasma exchange.

commonly seen in children. Short-term follow-up shows complete or nearly complete resolution of cord lesions, which distinguishes them from tumors such as glioneuronal neoplasias which may have a similar appearance.

Transverse myelitis

TM is a clinical syndrome with multiple etiologies. Imaging features include a long segment of involvement (usually 3–4 vertebral segments) and a large cross-sectional area of central cord signal abnormality, most commonly affecting the thoracic cord.[16] Enhancement is variable and is often present acutely.[21] Causes of TM include infection, systemic autoimmune or inflammatory disease, paraneoplastic syndrome, and postinfectious or postvaccination state (Fig. 7).[21]

In all these demyelinating and inflammatory lesions, the clinical presentation, extent, and pattern of cord involvement may help distinguish them from tumors. In addition, many of these lesions have skip involvement, with areas of abnormality separated by normal appearing cord, a finding that is uncommon with primary tumors but occasionally seen with metastases (spinal cord metastases however are extremely rare in children). Nearly all patients presenting with cord metastases are in the late course of their disease and have a definitive clinical history that aids in arriving at the correct imaging diagnosis.

Neurosarcoidosis

Spinal cord involvement in sarcoidosis is rare but important to consider in the differential of spinal cord tumor-like lesions, as occasionally it may be the first manifestation of the disease. Symptomatic neurosarcoidosis has been reported in 5% to 15% of patients with sarcoidosis. The prevalence of spinal sarcoidosis is not well studied but has been reported in less than 1% of all sarcoidosis patients.[22]

Common CNS findings include leptomeningeal enhancement (48%–67%) and enhancing intramedullary lesions (46%–100%).[22] Cord lesions are most often seen in the cervical region but occur anywhere along the cord. Long segments of involvement are most common, averaging 4.2 vertebral segments and with a predilection to affect the dorsal cord (Fig. 8).[22] Less commonly, lesions can be short and tumefactive and while the former is easily distinguished from tumors, the latter may pose difficulties.[23]

Various patterns of spinal involvement can be seen, likely due to different stages of the disease. Neurosarcoidosis is listed under intramedullary lesions in this article as this is the stage most likely to mimic a tumor. The stages have been classified by Junger and colleagues as follows:[24]

- Stage 1: linear leptomeningeal enhancement
- Stage 2: intramedullary enhancing lesion with cord enlargement

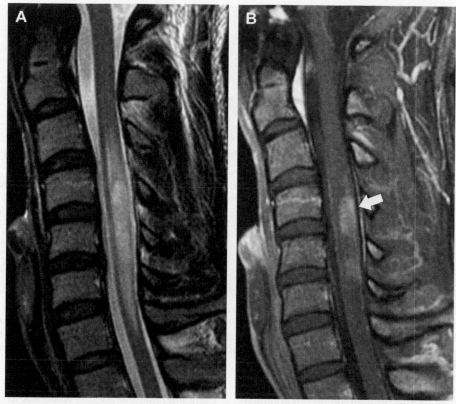

Fig. 7. Transverse myelitis. Sagittal T2WI (*A*) shows mildly expansile and heterogeneous signal abnormality involving the cervical cord. Sagittal post-contrast T1WI (*B*) shows patchy areas of contrast enhancement (*arrow*). Although distinguishing this appearance from neoplasm is difficult, as with ADEM, TM has an acute clinical onset and is responsive to steroids.

- Stage 3: normal-size cord with focal or multifocal enhancement
- Stage 4: cord atrophy and no enhancement

Differentiating sarcoidosis from tumors may be difficult, especially for those in stage 2, as patients with metastases or lymphoma may also have brain, lung, and other organs involved as does sarcoidosis. Sarcoidosis may occasionally show low T2 signal and somewhat restricted diffusion confusing it with lymphoma. In these instances, clinical and laboratory findings, including biopsy, may be required for a definitive diagnosis.

Infections

Infections within the spinal cord parenchyma are rare but should be considered in the presence of rapidly progressive neurological deficits, fever, and altered serum inflammatory markers.

A *bacterial spinal cord abscess* typically arises from adjacent osteomyelitis-discitis but may also occur due to hematogenous spread from other sources.[25] Imaging features are the same as

seen with a brain abscess, which includes a rim-enhancing lesion with central fluid that shows restricted diffusion.[25] Spinal cord abscesses are frequently associated with a large amount of edema for the size of the lesion (**Fig. 9**). Abscesses may have imaging features identical to metastases and lymphoma, but their clinical and laboratory findings help distinguish between them.

Another spinal infection to consider in the differential diagnosis of tumor-like lesions is a *tuberculoma*. These are caused by a granulomatous reaction to tuberculosis (TB) and arise from hematogenous dissemination. CNS TB is rare, accounting for approximately 0.5% to 2% of all cases, but has high mortality and morbidity, making early diagnosis crucial in improving outcomes. Early on, a tuberculoma causes severe inflammation and extensive cord edema with the homogenous enhancement of the TB lesion, and may be indistinguishable from primary and secondary tumors. As the internal gel content of the tuberculoma increases, T2WI may show alternating bands of low and high signal, described as the "target

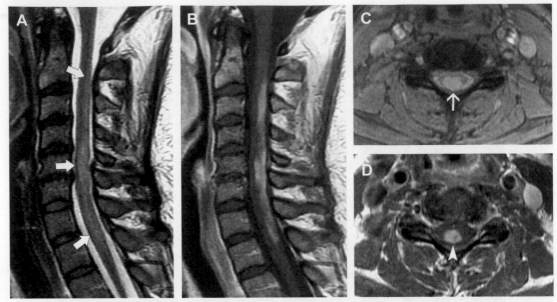

Fig. 8. Neurosarcoidosis. Sagittal T2WI (*A*) shows longitudinally extensive and mildly heterogeneous signal abnormality involving the cervical cord (*thick arrows*). Note a posterior predominant pattern of contrast enhancement (*B* and *D*, *arrowhead*). Axial T2* GRE (*C*) image shows near total involvement of the cross-section of the cord (*thin arrow*). The presence of cerebral, lung, and mediastinal lesions as well as patient's race should help suggest sarcoidosis. Also, sarcoidosis responds to steroids.

sign," as well as sharply marginated rim enhancement.[26] Of course, this latter finding is size dependent and may be absent in smaller lesions. Leptomeningeal disease is another common manifestation of spinal TB and can present with a nodular appearance, although any compartment may be affected (Fig. 10). Again, this pattern of pial involvement may be identical to that seen occasionally with metastases and lymphoma.

Neurosyphilis is rare but should be considered as a potential tumor mimic. A wide spectrum of intracranial and/or spinal imaging findings can be seen depending on its stage. In early neurosyphilis, meningitis can present with leptomeningeal enhancement and appear like bacterial or neoplastic meningitis, though neurosyphilis may appear more nodular. Mass-like and intramedullary syphilitic gummas can mimic a tumor.[27] Characterization of the imaging features of gummas is limited due to the rarity of this pathology. Yang and colleagues described some features including a hyperintense periphery with a hypointense-to-isointense central portion on T2WI and variable peripheral enhancement. Gummas can also be seen in the extramedullary and extradural spaces and mimic tumors.[27] Typical late-stage neurosyphilis findings include cerebral atrophy and tabes dorsalis. In the spinal cord, tabes dorsalis is seen as atrophy and hyperintense signal in the dorsal columns on T2WI, which can mimic subacute

combined degeneration.[28] Needless to say, syphilis is a difficult diagnosis, and the appearance of its lesions is non-specific, leading to a long differential diagnosis including tumors such as metastases and even intravascular lymphoma.

Cysticercosis, caused by *taenia solium*, affects the spine in about 5% of patients and the spinal cord in <1% of them. Cysticercosis tends to affect both genders equally especially in the 4th and 5th decades of life. Although the different stages of the disease are well known and help in the diagnosis of brain lesions, the findings in the spinal cord tend to be non-specific. Most lesions enhance and are accompanied by edema resulting in a broad differential diagnosis but occasionally, as in the brain, they may be cystic, show a scolex, and peripheral contrast enhancement which should suggest the diagnosis (Fig. 11).[29] Since 100% of patients have involvement elsewhere, imaging of brain and other organs may provide a clue to the diagnosis. More common than intramedullary cysticercosis is the extramedullary/intradural form. In this latter form, the lesions are in the subarachnoid space, tend to be cystic without a scolex, and may produce arachnoiditis often with accompanying inflammation of the nerve roots and even of the spinal cord.[30] Chronic arachnoiditis may result in tethering of the cord with intrinsic T2 signal changes and even syrinx formation. In addition, some patients show lesions in the spinal

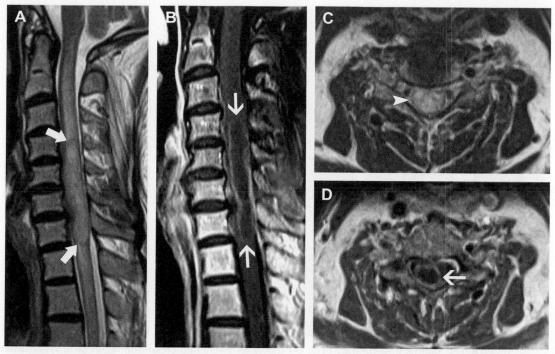

Fig. 9. Spinal cord abscess. Sagittal T2WI (*A*) shows an oblong mass-like lesion involving a long segment of the cervical cord (*thick arrows*) with extensive surrounding edema. Sagittal (*B*) and axial (*D*) post-contrast T1WI show peripheral ring-like enhancement (*thin arrows*). The lesion involves nearly the entire cross-section of the cord with little visible parenchyma (*C, arrowhead*). Features that help distinguish this lesion from tumor would be restricted diffusion (not shown) and clinically, a rapid progression, fever, and elevated serum inflammatory markers.

cord and simultaneously in the subarachnoid space. When cysticercosis is suspected, the most helpful finding is that of lesions in the brain which tend to be typical and suggest the diagnosis.[29,30] When the lesions show nonspecific patterns of contrast enhancement, the main differential diagnosis is metastases and in rare instances, metastases may also be cystic.

Among other parasitic diseases which rarely affect the spinal cord and result in cystic lesions is *echinococcus,* which predominantly occurs in the middle east, Turkey, and South America (Bolivia, Peru, and Chile). Its imaging findings are like those of cysticercosis, and diagnosis may be suggested if patients originated from or have traveled to endemic regions.[31,32] *Toxoplasmosis* may also involve the spinal cord especially in patients with malfunctioning immune systems. Unfortunately, its imaging findings are nonspecific, the diagnosis is difficult, and the main differential diagnosis is that of other infections and metastases.[33] *Schistosomiasis* may also rarely involve the cord. Because its clinical course is slower than that of other infections, it may be confused with neoplasia. It predominantly affects the conus

medullaris which shows diffuse contrast enhancement and edema, like that seen with infiltrating gliomas. However, schistosomiasis often results in inflammation of cauda equina, a finding that is not present in tumors. Schistosomiasis is relatively common in the Caribbean, Central, and South America as well as Southeast Asia and travel to these regions may suggest the diagnosis. Additionally, the disease has been linked to some sweet water lakes in Central Africa.[34]

Paraneoplastic Myelopathy

This rare condition represents an autoimmune disorder generally occurring in patients with underlying cancer. Most are female patients around 60 years of age. The clinical presentation is slow, with most symptoms increasing in a period of 3 to 4 weeks. Cancer of the breast, thymus, lung (small cell type), kidney, colon, ovary, testicles, and lymphoma can cause paraneoplastic myelopathy. In most of these patients, at least one neuronal antibody will be elevated confirming the diagnosis.[35] When a paraneoplastic myelopathy occurs without a primary tumor, a new search for

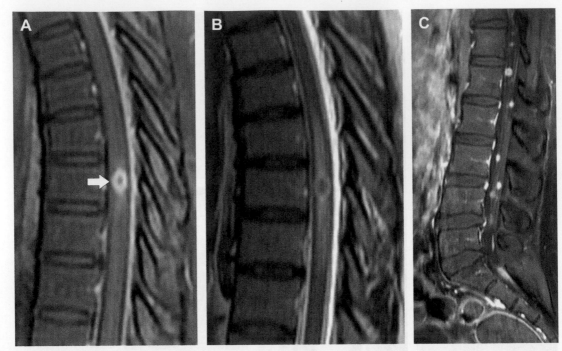

Fig. 10. Tuberculosis. Sagittal post-contrast T1WI (*A*) shows an avidly ring-enhancing lesion (*arrow*) consistent with a tuberculoma. Note surrounding edema on sagittal T2WI (*B*). Sagittal post-contrast T1WI in a different patient with leptomeningeal disease (*C*) shows numerous enhancing tuberculomas along the distal cord and cauda equina mimicking metastases or neurofibromas. (*Courtesy of* E Zamora, MD, Philadelphia, PA.)

a primary cause needs to be repeated 6 to 12 months after the diagnosis. MR imaging shows extensive intramedullary high T2 signal with non-specific contrast enhancement.[36] Involvement of the lateral and/or dorsal columns and the central gray matter should suggest the diagnosis and

differentiate it from metastases.[37] It should be noted that in symptomatic patients, up to 50% of them may have a normal MR imaging. The most important differential diagnoses include metastases, vitamin B12 deficiency, dAVF, sarcoidosis, and tuberculosis.

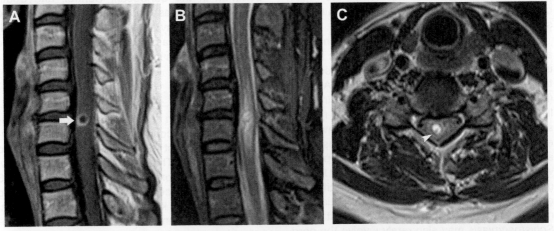

Fig. 11. Neurocysticercosis. Sagittal post-contrast T1WI (*A*) shows an intramedullary ring-enhancing lesion (*arrow*) with surrounding edema on the accompanying STIR sequence (*B*). A scolex is seen on the axial T2WI (*arrowhead, C*). Metastases can have a similar appearance, however, intramedullary metastases are rarely cystic and the presence of a scolex is typical of cysticercosis.

Intradural Extramedullary Lesions

There is a relatively limited differential for non-neoplastic intradural extramedullary lesions. These are often cystic-appearing lesions that may mimic a cystic neoplasm or distort the cord and cause edema that may be mistaken for an intramedullary tumor. Cystic-appearing lesions of the intradural extramedullary space can be congenital or acquired.

Arachnoid cysts and webs

While arachnoid webs are not true mass-like abnormalities, their effects on the spinal cord can mimic a tumor by distorting it and causing edema. Arachnoid cysts exert mass effect on the cord and can rarely be intramedullary. Since the webs or walls of the cysts are often imperceptible on conventional MR imaging sequences, these lesions are difficult to diagnose. High-resolution heavily T2-weighted sequences (T2 SPACE, FIESTA, CISS) help delineate the walls of the cyst or web. When present, these entities displace the cord to the opposite side of the thecal sac and may lead to edema, myelopathy, and occasionally syrinx formation.[38,39] Arachnoid cysts are most commonly seen dorsally in the thecal sac and follow CSF signal intensity on all MR imaging sequences. CT (Computed Tomography) myelography can help differentiate arachnoid cysts from spinal cord herniation as most cysts do not fill with contrast material initially and present as mass-like filling defects.[40,41] However, most cysts will eventually fill with contrast material, and some may exhibit rapid opacification and can be difficult to detect. Webs are primarily seen in the dorsal thoracic thecal sac. The focal dorsal indentation of the cord by a web has been described as the "scalpel sign" (Fig. 12).[42] Cord edema resulting from webs and cysts resolves soon after surgery. The cord T2 signal abnormality shows no contrast enhancement. The above MR imaging features clearly distinguish the associated cord abnormalities from tumors.

Spinal cord herniation

Like arachnoid webs, a spinal cord herniation is not a mass-like lesion but because it distorts the cord and can cause cord edema, it may be mistaken for a tumor. In herniations, the cord is anteriorly displaced, with complete loss of CSF ventral to it.[43] CT myelography and phase-contrast imaging are helpful in differentiating cord herniation from arachnoid cysts.[41] Phase-contrast imaging shows the absence of flow ventrally, due to the herniated cord, with normal CSF flow dorsally. In contrast, a dorsally located cyst will obstruct CSF flow posterior to the cord.[43] Cord edema induced by a herniation shows no contrast enhancement and resolves rapidly after surgery which helps distinguish it from masses.

Neurenteric cysts

These cysts are congenital, due to incomplete resorption of the neuroenteric canal and most often found in the thoracic region. The presence of a vertebral anomaly is a finding that can help differentiate a neurenteric cyst from other cystic lesions. These anomalies include Klippel-Feil syndrome, hemivertebra, butterfly vertebra, and scoliosis. Also, neurenteric cysts are usually ventral in location as opposed to the dorsal location of arachnoid cysts and webs. Neurenteric cysts can involve multiple compartments. On MR imaging, these cysts may have variable signal on T1 and T2 weighted images due to variations in protein contents (Fig. 13).[44,45] Like any compressive lesion, neuroenteric cysts may produce signal changes in the cord but the above-mentioned imaging features are typical and suggest the diagnosis.

Epidermoid cysts

Epidermoid cysts can be congenital or acquired. A congenital epidermoid is formed from inappropriate implantation of ectodermal cells within the neural tube during the closure, which occurs in the 3rd- 5th week of embryonic development.[46] These cysts are often associated with spinal malformations, including spinal dysraphisms and hemivertebrae.[47] An acquired epidermoid can rarely be the late complication of surgery or a lumbar puncture, and result from the implantation of epidermal elements in the spinal canal during the procedures.[48]

On imaging, congenital epidermoids are usually seen in the thoracic region, or near the cauda equina. Acquired epidermoids are typically seen in the lumbar region. MR imaging signal of spinal epidermoids varies depending on the content of water, lipids, and proteins within the cyst. Most commonly, epidermoids follow CSF signal intensity on T1WI and T2WI but are heterogeneously hyperintense on FLAIR and show restricted diffusion (Fig. 14). Usually, there is no contrast enhancement but a thin rim of enhancement is possible in some lesions and pronounced enhancement can be present with superimposed infection.[49] Infection also results in restricted diffusion. (41) Their imaging features are typical and should not be confused with true tumors. Occasionally, epidermoids and dermoids may coexist, and differentiating them from teratoma may not be possible.

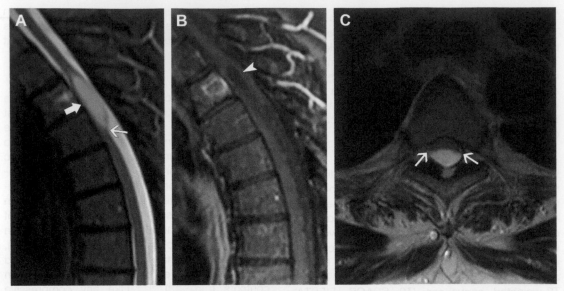

Fig. 12. Dorsal arachnoid web. Sagittal STIR (*A*) shows focal indentation of the dorsal cord consistent with a "scalpel sign" (*thin arrow*). There is abnormal cord signal above this level (*arrow*) due to a combination of edema and syrinx. Sagittal post-contrast T1WI (*B*) shows a focal hypointense structure within the cord corresponding to the syrinx. There is no contrast enhancement. Axial T2WI (*C*) shows marked flattening of the cord at the level of the indentation (*thin arrows*). Although the intramedullary expansile area may be confused with tumor, neoplasias do not have the "scalpel sign" which suggests the correct diagnosis.

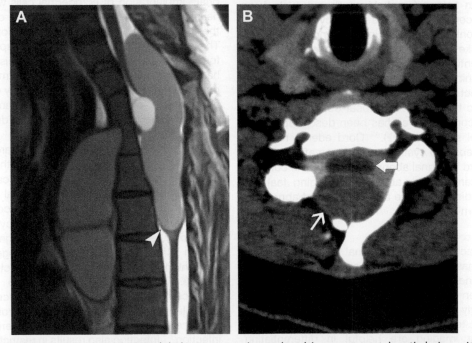

Fig. 13. Neurenteric cyst. Sagittal T2WI (*A*) shows a complex and multicompartmental cystic lesion with extradural, paraspinal, intradural, and intramedullary (*arrowhead*) components. Note dysplastic appearance of the vertebrae with segmentation anomalies. Axial CT myelography (*B*) shows a posterior filling defect corresponding to the cyst (*thin arrow*) with the mass effect on the cord (*thick arrow*). There is also a posterior fusion defect with the absence of the right lamina. Although the lesion does have an intramedullary component, the overall appearance suggests the correct diagnosis and distinguishes it from a neoplasia.

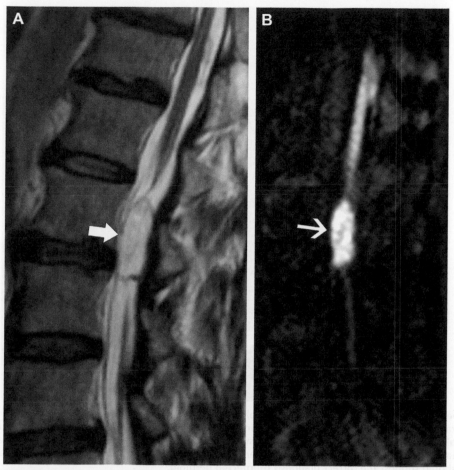

Fig. 14. Epidermoid. Sagittal T2WI (*A*) shows a bright ovoid mass along the filum terminale/cauda equina (*thick arrow*). There is prominent restricted diffusion on DWI (*thin arrow, B*). Although the differential diagnosis of this mass may include filar/cauda equina tumors such as ependymoma, neurofibroma, schwannoma, and others, the presence of significantly restricted diffusion and lack of enhancement (not shown) suggests the diagnosis of epidermoid.

Dermoid cysts

Spinal dermoids are similar to epidermoids but are thought to be solely congenital, and formed by the implantation of epithelial elements during neural tube closure.[50] Like epidermoid cysts, they are lined by stratified squamous epithelial cells, but contain dermal components, including sebaceous glands, sweat glands, hair follicles, and occasionally teeth.[50] On imaging, dermoids usually follow fat signal intensity with hyperintense signal on T1WI but are often heterogeneous due to the presence of other dermal components. This gives dermoids a heterogenous appearance on T2WI. Calcifications are also commonly seen.[50] Dermoids are less likely to show restricted diffusion as compared to epidermoids.[51] They are typically located in the

lumbosacral region and are extramedullary but are also seen along the cauda equina and not uncommonly can have intramedullary extension, especially in the conus medullaris.[51] When reviewing a case of a suspected dermoid cyst, it is important to look for signs of rupture, which will be seen as multiple T1 hyperintense foci disseminated in the subarachnoid space.[52] Most dermoids show no contrast enhancement, but as with epidermoids, enhancement can be present in infected lesions. The presence of a sinus tract increases the risk of infection (**Fig. 15**). Their lobulated, heterogenous signal, often with areas of high T1 signal intensity suggests the diagnosis. On occasion however, they may be indistinguishable from teratomas or even complex intraspinal lipomas.

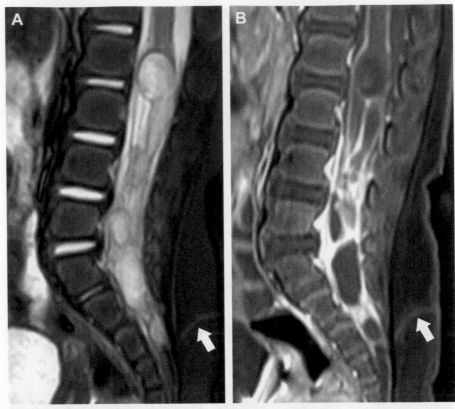

Fig. 15. Dermoid. Sagittal STIR (*A*) shows a complex multicystic lesion in the spinal canal. There is extensive post-contrast enhancement due to superimposed infection (*B*). Note sinus tract in the lower back (*arrows*). The differential diagnosis may include a tumor with distal metastases (atypical teratoid rhabdoid, malignant glioma, medulloblastoma, and so forth). The presence of areas with restricted diffusion (not shown) and the sinus tract however should suggest the correct diagnosis of infected dermoid.

Extradural Lesions

Extradural arachnoid cysts

Arachnoid cysts, previously discussed with intradural lesions, can also be seen in the extradural space. They can be congenital or acquired due to a dural defect that allows the arachnoid membrane to herniate beyond the dura and fill with CSF.[38] Their diagnosis is straightforward, but they may result in cord edema as seen in other compressive mass-like lesions. Synovial cysts should be included in the differential diagnosis of any extradural cyst; they tend to be lateral and located in proximity to an often degenerated facet joint.

Disc sequestrations

Disc herniation is a common finding in spinal imaging. These are usually easy to characterize but occasionally, they can have atypical signal, may be unusually large, or can become a free disc fragment that may be misinterpreted as a distinct lesion. A disc sequestration is defined as a disc extrusion that no longer has a connection to the parent disc.[53] The signal intensity can be variable depending on the age of the sequestration (**Fig. 16**).[54] Herniated discs may also be hemorrhagic, and these are generally T1 bright and must be differentiated from lesions such as neurenteric cysts, dermoids, and lipomas but more commonly, they need to be differentiated from tumors such as metastases and lymphoma which may show restricted diffusion and more homogeneous contrast enhancement.

Extramedullary hematopoiesis

Another extradural lesion to consider in the context of tumor-like lesions is extramedullary hematopoiesis. This is often seen as multiple enhancing paraspinal masses within the prevertebral or epidural space.[55] The lesions can have foci of fat signal intensity, suggesting non-active lesions (similar to yellow marrow), whereas enhancement and intermediate signal intensity are more likely to represent active hematopoietic lesions (similar to red marrow).[55] A helpful diagnostic finding is a diffusely

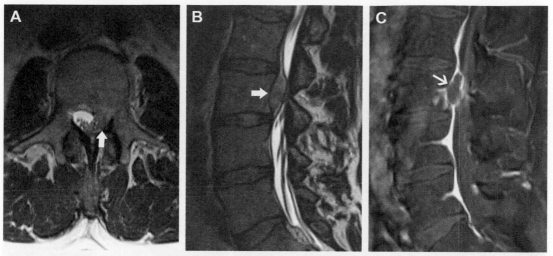

Fig. 16. Sequestered disc. Axial (*A*) and sagittal (*B*) T2WI show an isointense disc herniation arising from the L3-L4 disc, with cranial migration (*thick arrows*), and no attachment to the parent disc. There is effacement of the left subarticular zone and mass effect on the traversing nerve roots. Sagittal post-contrast T1WI (*C*) shows enhancement around the sequestered disc consistent with granulation tissue (*thin arrow*). The differential diagnosis for these lesions may include metastases, lymphoma, and even meningioma but peripheral contrast enhancement, lack of bone involvement, and acute symptoms should suggest the correct diagnosis.

decreased bone marrow signal intensity on T1 and T2 weighted sequences, suggesting underlying red marrow conversion. Some extramedullary lesions can be hypointense on both T1 and T2-weighted sequences due to iron deposition, particularly if there is a history of multiple blood transfusions (**Fig. 17**). Typically, patients with extramedullary hematopoiesis have known long-standing anemia (eg, thalassemia, sickle cell disease, hereditary spherocytosis) or a myeloproliferative disorder (eg, chronic myelogenous leukemia, polycythemia vera, essential thrombocytosis, myelofibrosis); or rarely diffuse osseous metastatic disease.[55–57] Severe cases of extramedullary hematopoiesis can cause spinal cord compression.[58]

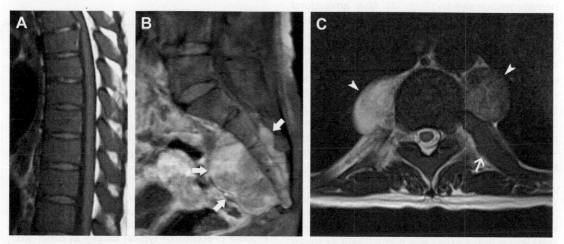

Fig. 17. Extramedullary hematopoiesis in a patient with beta thalassemia. Sagittal noncontrast T1WI (*A*) shows diffuse T1 hypointensity of the bone due to red marrow conversion (ie, bone marrow has lower signal intensity than the discs). Sagittal post-contrast T1WI (*B*) shows an enhancing mass arising from the inferior sacrum (*thick arrows*). Axial T2WI in a different patient (*C*) shows bilateral paraspinal masses with different signal intensities (*arrowheads*). Note associated rib expansion (*thin arrow*). The differential diagnosis includes metastases and lymphoma, but the expansion of the rib is unlikely with those 2 entities.

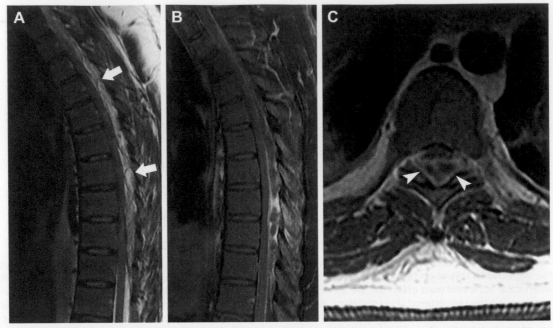

Fig. 18. Epidural abscess. Sagittal T2WI (*A*) shows an extensive heterogeneous lesion along the dorsal aspect of the spinal canal (*arrows*). Sagittal (*B*) and axial (*C*) post-contrast T1WI show extensive peripheral enhancement (*arrowheads* in *C*). Because there was no adjacent source of infection in the spine, this was presumed secondary to hematogenous spread. Lymphoma and rarely metastases may present with long epidural lesions. The former may also show restricted diffusion, but very rapidly developing symptoms, fever, and elevated serum inflammatory markers should help one suggest the diagnosis of epidural abscess.

Epidural abscess

An epidural abscess is usually not a diagnostic dilemma as they are commonly associated with adjacent discitis-osteomyelitis. However, occasionally, the adjacent infection may be less apparent, or they can present in isolation due to hematogenous seeding (**Fig. 18**). Also, an epidural abscess can sometimes be focal and appear as a rounded lesion. On imaging, an epidural abscess will have hyperintense signal on T2WI and demonstrate a thick rim of enhancement.[59,60] If DWI is obtained, this typically shows restricted diffusion within the non-enhancing central component, but this may be difficult to visualize as often epidural abscesses are small.[61] Epidural abscess may cause cord edema due to compression and venous thrombophlebitis with or without venous thrombosis.

SUMMARY

In this article, we have discussed multiple mass-like lesions in the spine that can present as tumor mimics. Some of them have characteristic imaging appearances that usually allow their differentiation from true neoplasms. Others have nonspecific and overlapping features that make them indistinguishable from primary or metastatic neoplasms

solely on the basis of imaging. For the latter group, patient's history, epidemiology, and clinical presentation are helpful to narrow the differential diagnosis.

CLINICS CARE POINTS

- Vascular lesions can be usually distinguished from neoplasms based on their characteristic imaging findings, however some tumors like paragangliomas can present with prominent vascularity.

- While restricted diffusion can be seen in cord infarction and lymphoma, an acute presentation, lack of contrast enhancement, and central cord involvement is consistent with infarction.

- Enhancing cord lesions in MS are rarely tumefactive and may be confused with neoplasia, however, an acute clinical presentation and the presence of typical lesions at other sites suggests MS.

- Large expansile lesions in NMO may simulate tumor but other characteristic imaging features along with clinical and laboratory findings help arrive at the correct diagnosis.

- While inflammatory lesions like ADEM and TM can present with an expansile appearance of the cord, they usually have an acute onset and are responsive to steroids, as opposed to neoplasia.
- Various lesions resulting from infection can simulate neoplasia and require correlation with the clinical presentation, epidemiology, and laboratory findings.
- Extramedullary lesions such as arachnoid webs can exert significant mass effect on the cord and mimic neoplasia if they result in significant cord edema.
- Epidermoids have characteristic MR imaging features but may have a complex appearance in the presence of superimposed infection and enhancement.
- Large disc extrusions and sequestered discs can occasionally simulate neoplasia, however, peripheral contrast enhancement, lack of osseous involvement, and acute symptoms should suggest the correct diagnosis.

DISCLOSURE

The authors have nothing to disclose.

REFERENCES

1. Kharkar S, Shuck J, Conway J, et al. The natural history of conservatively managed symptomatic intramedullary spinal cord cavernomas. Neurosurgery 2007;60(5):865–72. discussion 865-872.
2. Deutsch H, Jallo GI, Faktorovich A, et al. Spinal intramedullary cavernoma: clinical presentation and surgical outcome. J Neurosurg 2000;93(1 Suppl): 65–70.
3. Spetzger U, Gilsbach JM, Bertalanffy H. Cavernous angiomas of the spinal cord clinical presentation, surgical strategy, and postoperative results. Acta Neurochir 1995;134(3–4):200–6.
4. Mabray MC, Starcevich J, Hallstrom J, et al. High Prevalence of Spinal Cord Cavernous Malformations in the Familial Cerebral Cavernous Malformations Type 1 Cohort. AJNR Am J Neuroradiol 2020;41(6):1126–30.
5. Hegde AN, Mohan S, Lim CC. CNS cavernous haemangioma: "popcorn" in the brain and spinal cord. Clin Radiol 2012;67(4):380–8.
6. Turjman F, Joly D, Monnet O, et al. MRI of intramedullary cavernous haemangiomas. Neuroradiology 1995;37(4):297–302.
7. Ogilvy CS, Louis DN, Ojemann RG. Intramedullary cavernous angiomas of the spinal cord: clinical presentation, pathological features, and surgical management. Neurosurgery 1992;31(2):219–29. discussion 229-230.
8. Santoro A, Piccirilli M, Frati A, et al. Intramedullary spinal cord cavernous malformations: report of ten new cases. Neurosurg Rev 2004;27(2):93–8.
9. Morris JM. Imaging of dural arteriovenous fistula. Radiol Clin North Am 2012;50(4):823–39.
10. Krings T, Mull M, Gilsbach JM, et al. Spinal vascular malformations. Eur Radiol 2005;15(2):267–78.
11. Patsalides A, Knopman J, Santillan A, et al. Endovascular treatment of spinal arteriovenous lesions: beyond the dural fistula. AJNR Am J Neuroradiol 2011;32(5):798–808.
12. Masson C, Pruvo JP, Meder JF, et al. Spinal cord infarction: clinical and magnetic resonance imaging findings and short term outcome. J Neurol Neurosurg Psychiatry 2004;75(10):1431–5.
13. Ghosh PS, Mitra S. Owl's eye in spinal magnetic resonance imaging. Arch Neurol 2012;69(3):407–8.
14. Vargas MI, Gariani J, Sztajzel R, et al. Spinal cord ischemia: practical imaging tips, pearls, and pitfalls. AJNR Am J Neuroradiol 2015;36(5):825–30.
15. Yadav N, Pendharkar H, Kulkarni GB. Spinal Cord Infarction: Clinical and Radiological Features. J Stroke Cerebrovasc Dis 2018;27(10):2810–21.
16. Maj E, Wojtowicz K, Aleksandra, et al. Intramedullary spinal tumor-like lesions. Acta Radiol 2019;60(8): 994–1010.
17. Kandemirli SG, Reddy A, Hitchon P, et al. Intramedullary tumours and tumour mimics. Clin Radiol 2020;75(11):876 e817–e876 e832.
18. Sarbu N, Shih RY, Jones RV, et al. White Matter Diseases with Radiologic-Pathologic Correlation. Radiographics 2016;36(5):1426–47.
19. Yonezu T, Ito S, Mori M, et al. Bright spotty lesions" on spinal magnetic resonance imaging differentiate neuromyelitis optica from multiple sclerosis. Mult Scler 2014;20(3):331–7.
20. Mohajeri Moghaddam S, Bhatt AA. Location, length, and enhancement: systematic approach to differentiating intramedullary spinal cord lesions. Insights Imaging 2018;9(4):511–26.
21. Frohman EM, Wingerchuk DM. Clinical practice. Transverse myelitis. N Engl J Med 2010;363(6): 564–72.
22. Soni N, Bathla G, Pillenahalli Maheshwarappa R. Imaging findings in spinal sarcoidosis: a report of 18 cases and review of the current literature. NeuroRadiol J 2019;32(1):17–28.
23. Murphy OC, Salazar-Camelo A, Jimenez JA, et al. Clinical and MRI phenotypes of sarcoidosis-associated myelopathy. Neurol Neuroimmunol Neuroinflamm 2020;7(4):e722.
24. Junger SS, Stern BJ, Levine SR, et al. Intramedullary spinal sarcoidosis: clinical and magnetic resonance imaging characteristics. Neurology 1993;43(2): 333–7.
25. Takebe N, Iwasaki K, Hashikata H, et al. Intramedullary spinal cord abscess and subsequent

granuloma formation: a rare complication of vertebral osteomyelitis detected by diffusion-weighted magnetic resonance imaging. Neurosurg Focus 2014;37(2):E12.

26. Thirunavukarasu SC, Ramachandrappa A. A rare case of intramedullary tuberculoma: Complete resolution after medical treatment and role of magnetic resonance imaging in diagnosis and follow-up. Asian J Neurosurg 2012;7(4):223–6.

27. Yang C, Li G, Fang J, et al. Spinal Intramedullary Syphilitic Gumma: An Unusual Presentation of Neurosyphilis. World Neurosurg 2016;95:622 e617–e622 e623.

28. Pandey S. Magnetic resonance imaging of the spinal cord in a man with tabes dorsalis. J Spinal Cord Med 2011;34(6):609–11.

29. Leite CC, Jinkins JR, Escobar BE, et al. MR imaging of intramedullary and intradural-extramedullary spinal cysticercosis. AJR Am J Roentgenol 1997;169(6):1713–7.

30. Nash TE, O'Connell EM. Subarachnoid neurocysticercosis: emerging concepts and treatment. Curr Opin Infect Dis 2020;33(5):339–46.

31. Pamir MN, Ozduman K, Elmaci I. Spinal hydatid disease. Spinal Cord 2002;40(4):153–60.

32. Sioutis S, Reppas L, Bekos A, et al. Echinococcosis of the spine. EFORT Open Rev 2021;6(4):288–96.

33. Agrawal SR, Singh V, Ingale S, et al. Toxoplasmosis of spinal cord in acquired immunodeficiency syndrome patient presenting as paraparesis: a rare entity. J Glob Infect Dis 2014;6(4):178–81.

34. Joshi TN, Yamazaki MK, Zhao H, et al. Spinal schistosomiasis: differential diagnosis for acute paraparesis in a U.S. resident. J Spinal Cord Med 2010;33(3):256–60.

35. Passeri M, Matthews E, Kammeyer R, et al. Update in autoimmune and paraneoplastic myelopathies: Newly described antigen targets and antibody testing. Front Neurol 2022;13:972143.

36. Flanagan EP, McKeon A, Lennon VA, et al. Paraneoplastic isolated myelopathy: clinical course and neuroimaging clues. Neurology 2011;76(24):2089–95.

37. Shah S, Vazquez Do Campo R, Kumar N, et al. Paraneoplastic Myeloneuropathies: Clinical, Oncologic, and Serologic Accompaniments. Neurology 2021;96(4):e632–9.

38. Noujaim SE, Moreng KL, Noujaim DL. Cystic lesions in spinal imaging: a pictorial review and classification. Neurographics 2013;3(1):14–27.

39. Wenger M, Zobor N, Markwalder R, et al. Intradural extramedullary arachnoid cyst of the thoracic spine associated with cord compression. J Clin Neurosci 2007;14(7):693–6.

40. Khosla A, Wippold FJ 2nd. CT myelography and MR imaging of extramedullary cysts of the spinal canal in adult and pediatric patients. AJR Am J Roentgenol 2002;178(1):201–7.

41. Patel DM, Weinberg BD, Hoch MJ. CT Myelography: Clinical Indications and Imaging Findings. Radiographics 2020;40(2):470–84.

42. Reardon MA, Raghavan P, Carpenter-Bailey K, et al. Dorsal thoracic arachnoid web and the "scalpel sign": a distinct clinical-radiologic entity. AJNR Am J Neuroradiol 2013;34(5):1104–10.

43. Brugieres P, Malapert D, Adle-Biassette H, et al. Idiopathic spinal cord herniation: value of MR phase-contrast imaging. AJNR Am J Neuroradiol 1999;20(5):935–9.

44. Kemp SS, Towbin RB. Pediatric case of the day. Neurenteric cyst without associated vertebral anomalies. Radiographics 1992;12(6):1255–7.

45. Savage JJ, Casey JN, McNeill IT, et al. Neurenteric cysts of the spine. J Craniovertebr Junction Spine 2010;1(1):58–63.

46. Yousem DM, Grossman RI. Neuroradiology : the requisites. 3rd edition. Philadelphia, PA: Mosby/Elsevier; 2010.

47. Gonzalvo A, Hall N, McMahon JH, et al. Intramedullary spinal epidermoid cyst of the upper thoracic region. J Clin Neurosci 2009;16(1):142–4.

48. Beechar VB, Zinn PO, Heck KA, et al. Spinal Epidermoid Tumors: Case Report and Review of the Literature. Neurospine 2018;15(2):117–22.

49. Amato VG, Assietti R, Arienta C. Intramedullary epidermoid cyst: preoperative diagnosis and surgical management after MRI introduction. Case report and updating of the literature. J Neurosurg Sci 2002;46(3–4):122–6.

50. Messori A, Polonara G, Serio A, et al. Expanding experience with spontaneous dermoid rupture in the MRI era: diagnosis and follow-up. Eur J Radiol 2002;43(1):19–27.

51. Dahnert W. Radiology review manual. 7th Edition. Philadelphia: Wolters Kluwer Health/Lippincott Williams Wilkins; 2011.

52. Altay H, Kitis O, Calli C, et al. A spinal dermoid tumor that ruptured into the subarachnoidal space and syrinx cavity. Diagn Interv Radiol 2006;12(4):171–3.

53. Fardon DF, Williams AL, Dohring EJ, et al. Lumbar disc nomenclature: version 2.0: Recommendations of the combined task forces of the North American Spine Society, the American Society of Spine Radiology and the American Society of Neuroradiology. Spine J 2014;14(11):2525–45.

54. Konieczny MR, Reinhardt J, Prost M, et al. Signal Intensity of Lumbar Disc Herniations: Correlation With Age of Herniation for Extrusion, Protrusion, and Sequestration. Int J Spine Surg 2020;14(1):102–7.

55. Roberts AS, Shetty AS, Mellnick VM, et al. Extramedullary haematopoiesis: radiological imaging features. Clin Radiol 2016;71(9):807–14.

56. Choi H, David CL, Katz RL, et al. Case 69: extramedullary hematopoiesis. Radiology 2004;231(1):52–6.

57. Granjo E, Bauerle R, Sampaio R, et al. Extramedullary hematopoiesis in hereditary spherocytosis deficient in ankyrin: a case report. Int J Hematol 2002;76(2):153–6.

58. Lopes RRS, Cardoso LS, Onishi F. Spinal cord compression due to extramedullary hematopoiesis in beta-thalassemia. Arq Neuropsiquiatr 2020; 78(10):663–4.

59. Diehn FE. Imaging of spine infection. Radiol Clin North Am 2012;50(4):777–98.

60. Numaguchi Y, Rigamonti D, Rothman MI, et al. Spinal epidural abscess: evaluation with gadolinium-enhanced MR imaging. Radiographics 1993;13(3): 545–59. discussion 559-560.

61. Moritani T, Kim J, Capizzano AA, et al. Pyogenic and non-pyogenic spinal infections: emphasis on diffusion-weighted imaging for the detection of abscesses and pus collections. Br J Radiol 2014; 87(1041):20140011.

Imaging of Common and Infrequent Extradural Tumors

Andres Rodriguez, MD, Luis Nunez, MD,
David Timaran-Montenegro, MD, MSc, Roy Riascos, MD*

KEYWORDS

• Spine • Extradural tumor • Spinal tumor • Vertebral tumor

KEY POINTS

- Vertebral tumors might have an aggressive imaging appearance but benign behavior.
- Hemangiomas are the most common primary vertebral neoplasm and usually represent an incidental finding as most are asymptomatic.
- Osseous metastases represent the most common neoplasm of the spine, whereas primary extradural tumors constitute a smaller proportion of all spinal tumors.
- Multimodality imaging approach is often necessary to categorize primary bony lesions and delineate their soft tissue extension and associated complications.
- Magnetic resonance is the imaging modality of choice in detecting complications derived from extradural spine tumors.

INTRODUCTION

Spinal extradural (SE) tumors are uncommon lesions. However, patients with SE tumors have high morbidity and mortality. Imaging plays an essential role in establishing a differential diagnosis. Radiographs and computed tomography (CT) are the initial imaging modalities used for the assessment of symptomatic patients and to display the scope and characteristics of tumors. Key imaging features, such as type of matrix, cortical involvement, and margins, aid in the determination of a diagnosis. However, MR imaging is the preferred method for the assessment of SE tumors, as it allows for evaluation of complications that can increase morbidity, such as spinal cord and nerve compression, and invasion into the surrounding soft tissues and adjacent organs. This article discusses common and infrequent extradural spinal neoplasms and their imaging characteristics.

Enostosis

Enostosis, or bone islands, are incidental and asymptomatic lesions occurring in patients of all ages, with a propensity to involve the axial skeleton, especially the vertebral bodies, the ribs, and the pelvis. Usually, most lesions remain stable; however, some can slowly increase in size.[1]

This tumor appears as round lesion located adjacent to the endosteal surface of the cortex, with a size range between 2 and 20 mm and an irregular and spiculated margin that blends into the surrounding cancellous bone.[2] On x-rays and CT, enostosis are focal lesions with homogenous high-density and brushed borders at the periphery (Fig. 1). On MR imaging, they show low signal intensity on T1 and T2-weighted images (T2WI), with no adjacent bone marrow abnormality. No bone destruction, periosteal reaction, soft tissue involvement, or increase in the size greater than 25% should be seen in a period of 6 months.

Department of Diagnostic and Interventional Imaging, The University of Texas Health Science Center at Houston, McGovern Medical School, 6431 Fannin Street MSB 2130B, Houston, TX 77030, USA
* Corresponding author.
E-mail address: Roy.F.Riascos@uth.tmc.edu

Neuroimag Clin N Am 33 (2023) 443–457
https://doi.org/10.1016/j.nic.2023.03.004
1052-5149/23/© 2023 Elsevier Inc. All rights reserved.

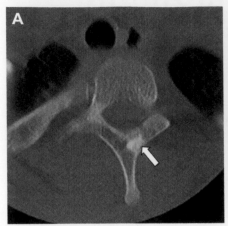
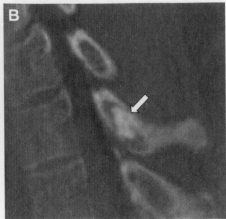

Fig. 1. Enostosis. CT axial (*A*) and sagittal (*B*) images show a homogenous hyperdense lesion with spiculated margins, adjacent to the cortex of the spinolaminar region (*arrows*). There is no associated cortical involvement, bone destruction, or periosteal reaction.

The absence of any of these findings suggests an alternate diagnosis, and a biopsy should be considered (Table 1).[2,3]

Osteoid Osteoma

Osteoid osteomas account for approximately 10% to 25% of spinal bone tumors, with a higher prevalence in males and a peak incidence during the second decade. Osteoid osteomas share similar histological findings with osteoblastomas; the main difference between the two entities being primarily the size, as osteoid osteomas measure less than 20 mm.[4,5]

Osteoid osteomas are considered benign lesions, generally involving the posterior elements, with a propensity for the lumbar spine. Clinical presentation of night back pain relieved by nonsteroidal anti-inflammatory drugs (NSAIDs) is representative of this lesion. Pain is presumed to be secondary to nerve innervation at the nidus, which is stimulated by vascular pressure and production of prostaglandins, thus explaining the

ability of NSAIDs to relieve it. Painful scoliosis secondary to muscle spasm is another common clinical finding, induced by inflammation related to the tumor, and radicular pain with gait disturbance.[4,6,7]

Diagnosing osteoid osteomas with x-rays may be challenging, given the small size of the lesion (<1.5 cm), its location in the posterior elements, and the spine anatomy that obscures the radiolucent nidus. They appear as a radiolucent lesion with reactive sclerosis, with or without a visible nidus. CT is considered the preferred method to characterize these lesions and usually demonstrates a well-defined soft tissue attenuating nidus, with a central and variable grade of mineralization. The nidus generally enhances with contrast, and serpentine or linear grooves may be seen around the lesion, representing enlarged arterioles. Enlarged arterioles are a highly specific finding for osteoid osteomas. MR imaging findings are variable and likely related to the degree of mineralization, usually seen as a low to intermediate signal on T1WI and intermediate signal on T2WI. Perilesional edema is common and can obscure the nidus, simulating a more aggressive lesion. Post-contrast images show avid enhancement secondary to the vascularity of these lesions (Fig. 2, Table 2).[2,5,8]

Osteoblastoma

Osteoblastomas are rare lesions that share similar histologic characteristics with osteoid osteomas; however, they are distinct based on their clinical course and radiologic findings. They generally manifest in the second decade of life, with a male predominance. Patients might be

Table 1		
Comparison of enostosis and metastasis in MR imaging findings		
Imaging Characteristic	Enostosis	Metastasis
Borders	Spiculated	Round
Bone destruction	None	May occur
Size	Stable	May increase in size
Number	Usually single	Single/multiple

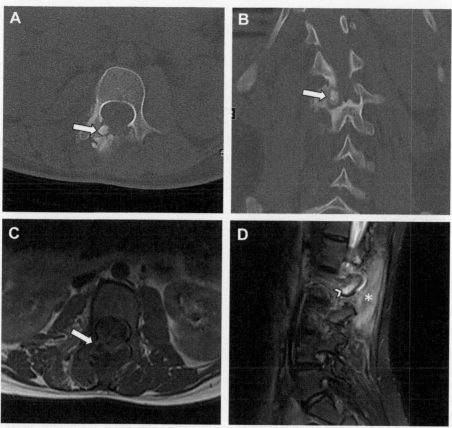

Fig. 2. Osteoid osteoma. Axial (*A*) and coronal (*B*) CT images show a lucent nidus surrounded by sclerosis in the right lamina with central calcification. Note that there is left convexity scoliosis with the vertex centered at the level of the lesion. T1WI (*C*) demonstrates a central hypointense calcification (*arrow*) with surrounding intermediate signal corresponding to the noncalcified nidus. Sagittal STIR (*D*) shows bone marrow edema involving the posterior elements and the vertebral body (*arrowhead*) and edema of the surrounding paraspinal soft tissues (*asterisk*).

asymptomatic, though they can present with constant dull pain with neurologic symptoms due to the local aggressiveness of some of the lesions that may compromise the adjacent neural structures. Osteoblastomas originate in the posterior elements and some extend into the vertebral body with equal predominance in the cervical, thoracic, and lumbar spine.[8]

Osteoblastomas are seen in radiography as solitary lesions with well-defined and usually lobulated margins. A sclerotic rim is seen in a proportion of osteoblastomas but is less common than osteoid osteomas. Three imaging patterns have been described on CT. The first is a mass with a central soft tissue density and surrounding sclerotic rim, similar to the classical appearance of osteoid osteoma, however, with a size greater than 20 mm. The second is an expansile mass with small calcifications and a sclerotic rim. The third and most common pattern is a locally

aggressive mass with mixed matrix that may invade soft tissues and cause bone destruction.[2,7] Osteoblastomas do not have a specific MR imaging pattern. Generally, they are hypointense on T1WI with a variable signal on T2WI and enhancement on post-contrast images. Nevertheless, MR imaging is useful in evaluating the involvement of adjacent soft tissues, nerve roots, and potential spinal cord compression (see **Table 2**).[4]

Giant Cell Tumor

Giant cell tumors (GCTs) are tumors generally centered in the appendicular bones with approximately 7% to 15% of the cases occurring in the spine mainly in the sacrum. This is opposite to the majority of primary spinal bone tumors that have a predilection for the vertebral bodies and may extend into the posterior elements. There is a slight predilection for females with a peak

Table 2
Comparison of osteoid osteoma and osteoblastomas

	Osteoid Osteoma	Osteoblastoma
Size	<1.5 cm	>1.5 cm
Local invasion	Confined	Soft tissue extension
Malignant degeneration	None/regression	Potential for malignant degeneration
Pain	Night	Dull constant/asymptomatic
Scoliosis	More common	Less common
Neurologic symptoms	Less common	More common
Location	Neural arch	Neural arch extending to vertebral body
Bone marrow edema	extensive	Less extensive

presentation during the second to fourth decades, being rare before skeletal maturity has been accomplished. An increase in size can be seen during pregnancy secondary to hormonal stimulation. Pain is the predominant symptom at presentation with an average duration of 5 months before diagnosis. Radicular pain and neurologic deficit might also be present.[2,9,10]

GCTs are benign but locally aggressive. These tumors contain areas histologically similar to an aneurysmal bone cyst (ABC); thus, imaging and proper biopsy specimen should be obtained to avoid diagnostic misinterpretation.[11,12]

Radiographs and CT show an osteolytic expansile lesion with no mineralization that has a narrow transition zone and usually invades the cortex. These lesions can demonstrate invasion of the sacroiliac joints, destruction of the foramina, and can cross the midline in the sacrum. The involvement of intervertebral discs and adjacent soft tissue may occur, simulating an infectious process. On MR imaging, they show low to intermediate signal on T1WI and T2WI. Contrast is helpful in evaluating soft tissue and epidural extension, as heterogeneous contrast enhancement is visualized in these lesions. Hemorrhagic areas are hyperintense on T1WI (**Fig. 3**). A CT-guided biopsy is recommended with a core needle. Fine needle biopsy of the bone and fluid-fluid levels should be avoided, as osteoclastic giant cells may be similar to Paget's disease on fine needle aspirations and fluid-fluid levels could represent ABC-like changes that do not harbor diagnostic tissue.[1,4,11]

Aneurysmal Bone Cyst

ABCs are considered true neoplasms. The name corresponds to a descriptive term for the lesion due to its pathologic appearance of distended fluid cavities. ABCs account for approximately 1% of bone tumors with 8% to 30% of the cases occurring in the spine, constituting approximately 15% of all primary spine tumors. There is a slight predilection for the cervical spine (40%), followed by the thoracic and lumbar spine. ABC is predominant in the pediatric population with an equal female-to-male ratio.[13,14]

In the 2020 World Health Organization Classification of Bone Tumors, the new nomenclature classifies these lesions as ABC and ABC-like changes, the latter commonly associated with GCT and chondroblastoma. ABCs are benign tumors composed of cystic cavities filled with blood.[14,15]

In radiographs, ABCs show an expansile mass that remodels the bone with a thin contour, generally centered in the posterior elements with a frequent involvement of the vertebral body. CT shows multiple cystic lesions with fluid–fluid levels that are highly sensitive and specific for ABCs. This lesion does not contain a matrix, and in most cases, there is an uninterrupted cortical bone at the lesion's periphery. MR imaging shows multiple cystic lesions with fluid–fluid levels and hemorrhagic components. Peripheral low signal on T1WI and T2WI represents the periosteum or pseudocapsule. Short Tau Inversion Recovery (STIR) images show subtle edema, and contrast images depict an enhancing septum (**Fig. 4**).[4,13]

Osteochondroma

Osteochondromas are considered the most common benign bone tumor, also called exostoses.[16] They are pedunculated lesions covered by a fibrous perichondrium or cartilaginous cap. Osteochondromas are usually found in the appendicular skeleton with 1% to 4% of the lesions presenting in the spine and a higher incidence in hereditary

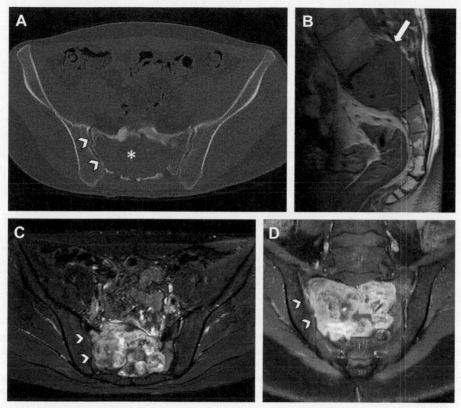

Fig. 3. GCT. Axial CT (*A*) image shows an expansile lytic mass with no matrix centered on the sacrum, extending into the sacral wings (*asterisk*, predominantly on the right side). There is no involvement of the lateral sacral cortex, and the right sacroiliac joint is preserved (*arrowheads*). Sagittal T1WI (*B*) image shows a hypointense mass that extends into the epidural space, occupying part of the sacral canal (*arrow*). On axial STIR image (*C*), the mass is predominantly hyperintense with some areas of hypointensity, and on coronal post-contrast T1WI (*D*), there is heterogenous enhancement.

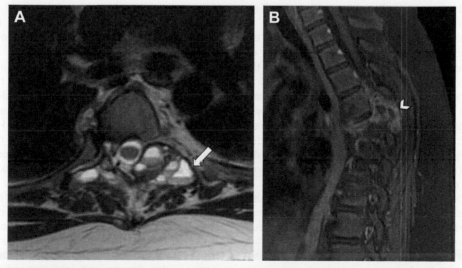

Fig. 4. ABC. Axial T2WI (*A*) image shows a multicystic mass centered in the posterior elements of a thoracic vertebra with fluid–fluid levels corresponding to hemorrhagic components (*arrow*). The septa demonstrate peripheral enhancement on sagittal post-contrast T1WI (*arrowhead* in *B*).

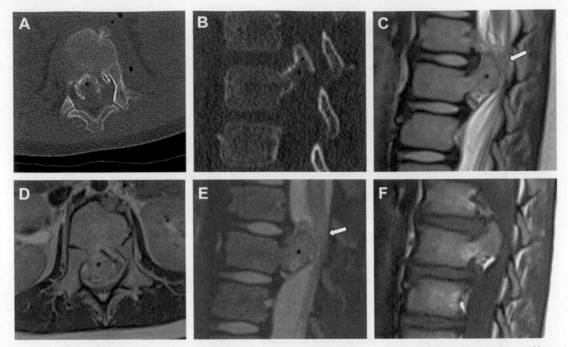

Fig. 5. Osteochondroma. Axial (*A*) and sagittal (*B*) CT images demonstrate an exophytic bony lesion (*asterisk*) protruding into the spinal canal with moderate spinal canal stenosis. MR imaging sagittal T2WI (*C*), axial T2WI (*D*), sagittal STIR (*E*), and sagittal T1WI (*F*) confirm the exophytic bony origin. The lesion (*asterisk*) is continuous with the posterior wall of the vertebral body and follows similar signal characteristics as the vertebral body on all sequences. There is severe compression and flattening of the conus medullaris and cauda equina nerve roots (*white arrows* in *C* and *E*).

cases. The cervical spine is the most commonly affected segment (50%), believed to be secondary to microtrauma due to cervical spine mobility that affects the cartilage growth plate. Exostoses can be solitary lesions or seen in hereditary multiple exostoses (HME), an autosomal dominant disease linked to a mutation in the existing genes that should be suspected with multiple osteochondromas.[17,18]

There is a male predominance, and most are diagnosed under the age of 20 years. Posterior elements are more commonly affected due to the position of ossification centers in this location. Symptoms usually present during adulthood, secondary to compression of adjacent structures with most cases being asymptomatic due to outward growing from the posterior elements. Histologically, there is no difference between solitary or HME, seen as a lesion with central lamellar bone covered by a cap of hyaline cartilage.[16,17,19]

On radiographs, osteochondromas are usually occult lesions. On CT, however, an excrescence demonstrating a direct continuity with the marrow and cortex from the parent bone is seen, which is highly pathognomonic of these lesions. MR imaging is useful for follow-up, which shows similar signal intensity to the originating bone with a cartilage cap that is iso- to hypointense on T1WI and

hyperintense on T2WI. A cartilage cap that exceeds 1.5 mm of thickness must raise the suspicion of malignant transformation to chondrosarcoma (**Fig. 5**).[2,9,19]

Hemangiomas

Hemangiomas are considered the most common benign vertebral neoplasms; however, these lesions are not true neoplasms, but rather venous malformations. The thoracic spine is most commonly affected but can occur at any spine level. Lesions are generally centered on the vertebral body and may extend into the posterior elements with the epidural and paraspinal spaces involved in aggressive hemangiomas. Hemangiomas are typically discovered between the fourth and fifth decade and have no sex predominance; 25% to 30% of these lesions are multiple. Hemangiomas are usually asymptomatic, whereas expansive lesions termed aggressive hemangiomas present symptoms due to neural compression, vertebral fracture, or cortical erosion.[20]

Hemangiomas have a dysembryogenic origin representing a hamartomatous lesion.[21] The nonvascular component includes adipose tissue, smooth muscle, fibrous tissue, bone, or hemosiderin.[22]

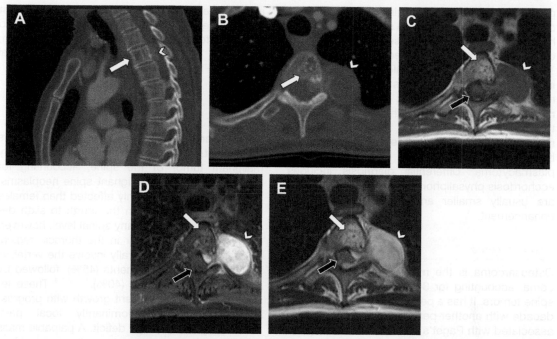

Fig. 6. Hemangioma. Sagittal (*A*) and axial (*B*) CT images show a heterogeneous predominantly lucent lesion with multiple dense trabeculae involving the T3 vertebral body (*arrows*). Note the soft tissue component extending to the epidural and paravertebral spaces (*arrowheads*). Axial T1WI, STIR, and post-contrast T1WI (*C–E*) show hyperintensity of the bone lesion on T2WI with suppression on STIR due to the fatty component (*white arrows*). Multiple hypointense intralesional dots represent the trabeculae. An enhancing paraspinal and epidural soft tissue component (*arrowheads*) displaces the spinal cord (*black arrows*).

Radiography shows coarse trabeculae within the lesion, described as a "corduroy" sign. CT, as in radiographs, shows coarse vertical hyperdense trabeculae that are seen as multiple sclerotic dots in axial images, creating the polka dot sign. On MR imaging, these lesions demonstrate increased signal on T1WI and T2WI with saturation on STIR images due to the fatty component that is typical in hemangiomas. Owing to its vascular component, enhancement is commonly seen. Imaging features that suggest a more aggressive behavior include a soft tissue component, whole vertebral body compromise, extension to the pedicles, bony expansion, cortical involvement, invasion of the epidural space or paraspinal space, and cord or nerve compression (Fig. 6).[2,4,23]

Chordoma

Chordomas are rare tumors and account for 2% to 4% of all malignant bone tumors. It is, however, the most common malignant tumor of the sacrum and the most common primary malignant tumor of the spine. It originates from notochordal remnants. During embryological development, notochordal cells involute along the vertebral column. However, some remnants stay along the spine, some remain

dormant, and others may evolve into chordomas.[24] Fifty percent are located in the sacrum and 10% to 15% in the vertebral bodies. The average age of diagnosis is between the fifth and seventh decades with a similar incidence between males and females.[25] They are considered slow-growing sarcomas and usually confined, locally aggressive in 20% of cases, and metastatic in 7%. Tumors arising from the sacrum are generally larger than the clivus and mobile spine. The main treatment of these lesions is surgical due to inadequate response to radiotherapy and chemotherapy.[26]

Macroscopically, chordomas are a multilobulated solid tumor with a gelatinous appearance. Histology shows epithelioid cells with bubbly cytoplasm called physaliphorous cells. The chondroid chordoma variant shows a myxoid matrix with hyaline cartilage features, resembling a chondrosarcoma.[27]

The radiograph may be normal in small lesions or might show a large mixed lytic and sclerotic lesion with soft tissue mass. CT demonstrates a lytic lesion with a lobulated soft tissue component that generally is more prominent anteriorly. Calcified foci are frequently seen. MR imaging in sacral involvement shows bone marrow replacement with soft tissue mass that might extend to the presacral space. On MR imaging, this tumor demonstrates low to intermediate signal on T1WI and high signal on T2WI representing the myxoid component and heterogeneous enhancement. The involvement of the mobile spine has similar intrinsic MR imaging findings as sacral involvement. In the mobile spine, it is common to see multiple-level involvement with a paraspinal mass that spares the disc (**Fig. 7**). Vertebral bone marrow replacement can resemble the "pseudobrain" appearance that has been described in plasmacytoma. Differential diagnosis includes ecchordosis physaliphora. These lesions however are usually smaller and have minimal or no enhancement.[24]

Osteosarcoma

Osteosarcoma is the most common spine sarcoma, accounting for 3% to 15% of all primary spine tumors. It has a peak incidence in the fourth decade with another peak in the seventh decade associated with Paget's disease. Osteosarcomas demonstrate a male predominance and are commonly found along the posterior elements of the thoracic and lumbar spine. This tumor presents with pain and a palpable mass with neurological deficit in 70% to 80% of the cases. Most of the times, it involves a single spinal level, and alkaline phosphatase is generally elevated due to increased bone turnover.[2,4,28]

Osteosarcomas have different histological subtypes, each with a variable osteoid matrix. Classification is established on the predominant type of extramedullary matrix, in which imaging correlation plays a central role.[28]

Radiographs show a destructive lesion with cortical involvement and a wide zone of transition. Mineralization matrix is generally seen. CT gives better visualization of the matrix, which can be obscured by contrast media. MR imaging findings

are variable and depend on the subtype. Contrast enhancement is usually heterogeneous and essential for evaluating soft tissue extension, especially into the spinal canal and neural foramina (**Fig. 8**).[4]

Chondrosarcoma

Chondrosarcomas are malignant cartilage tumors and constitute the second most common primary malignant tumor of the spine, accounting for 25% of the primary malignant spine neoplasms. Males are more commonly affected than females with a peak incidence in the fourth to sixth decades. They may affect any spinal level; however, 60% of the cases occur in the thoracic region. Chondrosarcomas generally involve the vertebral body and posterior elements (45%), followed by posterior elements only (40%).[10,29,30] These lesions usually have indolent growth with progressive symptoms, predominantly focal pain, followed by a neurologic deficit. A palpable mass in the back is common as it usually compromises the posterior elements. Histology shows a mesenchymal tumor with a cartilaginous appearance of unclear cell origin.[29,31]

Radiographs show a destructive bone mass with chondroid mineralization. CT demonstrates similar findings as radiographs with an expansile soft tissue mass usually centered in the posterior elements that displays bony erosions and chondroid matrix. As the lesion progresses in grade, there is less chondroid matrix and more myxoid component. MR imaging is useful for evaluating the soft tissue component. Generally, these lesions show low to intermediate T1WI signal and high signal on T2WI due to unmineralized cartilage with high water content. Post-contrast images show moderate to intense heterogenous enhancement[31] (**Fig. 9**).

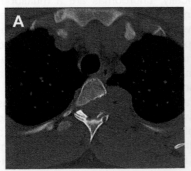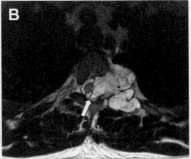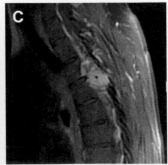

Fig. 7. Chordoma. Axial (*A*) CT image shows a left soft tissue attenuating pedicular mass with no matrix (*asterisk*). Axial T2WI (*B*) and sagittal post-contrast T1WI (*C*) show a T2 bright, enhancing mass with bubbly appearance (*asterisk*) that invades the epidural space and compresses the spinal cord (*arrow* in *B*).

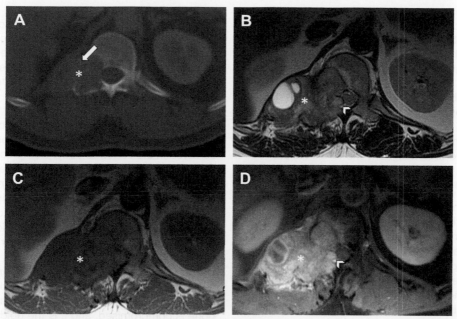

Fig. 8. Osteosarcoma. Axial CT image (*A*) shows an aggressive lytic mass involving the right posterior elements of a thoracic vertebra, extending into the vertebral body, paraspinal soft tissues, and costovertebral joint (*asterisk*). There are some dotted-like calcifications representing an osteoid matrix (*arrow*). Axial T2WI (*B*) demonstrates areas of cystic degeneration and epidural extension displacing the spinal cord (*arrowheads* in *B* and *D*). The mass (*asterisk* in *B–D*) is hypointense on T1WI (*C*), and demonstrates diffuse and ill-defined enhancement on T1WI post-contrast (*D*).

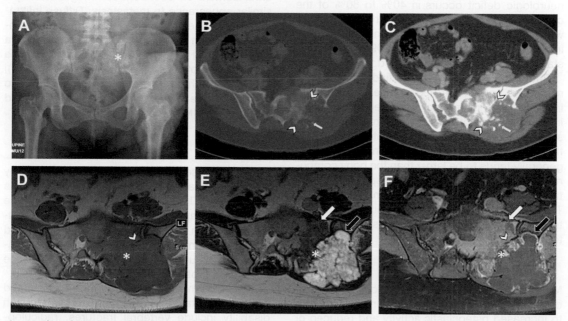

Fig. 9. Chondrosarcoma. Pelvic x-ray (*A*) shows an expansile ill-defined osteolytic mass involving the left sacral wing and adjacent iliac bone (*asterisk*). Axial CT images in bone (*B*) and soft tissue (*C*) window show an osteolytic mass with a chondroid matrix (*yellow arrows*) and sacroiliac joint involvement (*arrowheads*). Axial T1WI (*D*) and T2WI (*E*) demonstrate a T1 diffusely hypointense mass with bright T2 signal in the chondroid component (*black arrow* in *E*), and a solid component (*white arrow* in *E*), there is extension into the left sacroiliac joint (*asterisk* in *D*, *E*, *F*) with some cortical sacral bone preserved (*arrowheads* in *D*, *F*). Axial TIWI post-contrast (*F*) shows diffuse enhancement of the solid component (*white arrow* in *F*), and peripheral enhancement on the chondroid component (*black arrow* in *F*).

Chordoma should be considered in the differential diagnosis. Chordomas however always involve the vertebral body without involvement of the intervertebral vertebral disc, whereas chondrosarcomas have the propensity to involve the posterior elements and the vertebral body and can invade the vertebral disc. Benign cartilaginous lesions such as osteochondromas can simulate chondrosarcoma. When the cartilaginous cap of osteochondromas is greater than 2 cm thick, it is suggestive of a malignant chondroid lesion.[31]

Ewing Sarcoma

Ewing sarcoma (ES) is a rare primary spinal tumor, representing around 3% to 10% of all ES. It is the most common primary malignant spine bone tumor in patients less than 35 year old. There is a predilection for males with most tumors diagnosed before the third decade. The sacrum is involved in 55% of the cases, followed by the lumbar spine in 25%. ES is generally centered in the posterior elements and may extend into the vertebral body. Extraskeletal spinal ES can involve the paraspinal musculature with invasion into the epidural space.[10,32]

Localized pain is the most common presenting symptom and may be associated with fever, leukocytosis, or elevated sedimentation rate. A neurologic deficit occurs in 40% to 60% of the cases. Histology consists of small, round blue cells with an oval nucleus. The diagnosis relies on immunohistochemistry, with CD99 and Mic2 stains being most commonly used.[28]

Radiographs have variable findings and can mimic the permeative appearance of osteomyelitis. Vertebra plana may be seen. CT images improve radiograph findings and show large paraspinal masses that contain no matrix and invade the epidural space. The paraspinal component generally tends to be larger than the bony component. MR imaging findings are nonspecific, and the tumor is usually of intermediate signal on T1WI and T2WI (Fig. 10). The extraosseous component tends to be homogeneous in all sequences due to the lack of matrix.[4,10]

Multiple Myeloma

Multiple myeloma (MM) is a monoclonal plasma cell proliferative disorder in the bone marrow due to increased osteoclastic activity and reduced or suppressed osteoblastic function that leads to osteoporosis and osteolytic lesions.[33] It is the second most common hematologic malignancy after non-Hodgkin's lymphoma. It is a disorder seen in older adults with a peak of presentation in the seventh decade.[34] Imaging is essential to identify

bone lesions, start treatment early, and for follow-up. On the other hand, plasmacytoma is considered a solitary lesion in the absence of other features of MM.[33,35] The spine is the predominant area of compromise in MM with a preference for the vertebral bodies. Symptoms include fatigue, bone pain, and recurrent infections.[4,34]

Radiography may be normal in 20% of the cases and has poor sensitivity in detecting lesions. It can show a well-circumscribed lytic lesion usually centered in the vertebral body. Compression fractures are a common finding and might be the initial presentation. Osteopenia is almost invariably present in all cases. CT shows similar findings to x-rays with a more accurate depiction of MM lesions. It allows better definition of lytic lesions, fractures, cortical involvement, and extraosseous component, aiding to identify areas of instability with an elevated risk of fracture. MR imaging is the best imaging modality for diagnosis, follow-up, and for evaluation before the mineralized bone is compromised, and it is the gold standard for bone marrow assessment.[4,35] Different patterns have been described in MR imaging. Owing to the high fatty component in the bone marrow at the age of presentation, MM lesions might be seen as focal and hypointense on T1WI with intermediate to high signal on T2WI and STIR and enhancement on post-contrast images having a similar appearance to metastasis. Diffuse infiltration of the bone marrow is seen as diffuse hypointense signal on T1WI. A mixed pattern is seen as a combination of focal and diffuse lesions, giving the appearance of "salt and pepper" (Fig. 11). Diffusion-weighted images (DWI) have shown to be a sensitive sequence in the detection and follow-up of MM lesions.[34–36]

Metastases

Bone is a frequent site for metastases, followed by lung and liver, and affects up to 10% of all patients with cancer. The spine is the most common site involved with approximately 60% of bone metastases found in this location due to the high red marrow content in the vertebrae. The most common primary tumors that metastasize to the spine are breast, prostate, and lung[37,38] (Fig. 12).

Pain is the most common symptom associated with spine metastases. Symptoms related to high disability include vertebral fractures, radiculopathy, and in approximately 10% of cases, cord compression. Other symptoms related to bone resorption are secondary to hypercalcemia, such as constipation, fatigue, and cardiac arrhythmia. Imaging plays a crucial role in timely detection and thus early management which allows for

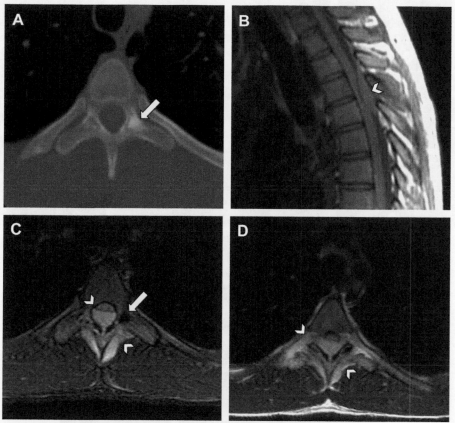

Fig. 10. Ewing's sarcoma. CT image (*A*) shows a well-defined osteoblastic lesion in the left pedicle (*arrow*). Sagittal T1WI (*B*) and axial T2WI with fat saturation (*C*) demonstrate the left pedicular osteoblastic lesion on T2WI (*arrow*) with adjacent paraspinal and epidural mass that compresses the spinal cord (*arrowheads*). The epidural and paraspinal mass show homogenous enhancement in the T1WI post-contrast (*arrowheads* in *D*).

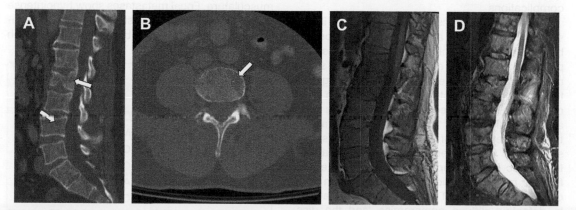

Fig. 11. Multiple myeloma. Sagittal (*A*) and axial (*B*) CT images show diffuse osteopenia with multiple well-defined punched-out lytic lesions involving multiple levels (*arrows*). There is an L2 pathologic fracture. Sagittal T1WI (*C*) demonstrates diffusely decreased marrow signal and sagittal T2WI (*D*) shows a speckled "salt and pepper" bone marrow appearance, secondary to diffuse and focal compromise of the bone marrow, respectively.

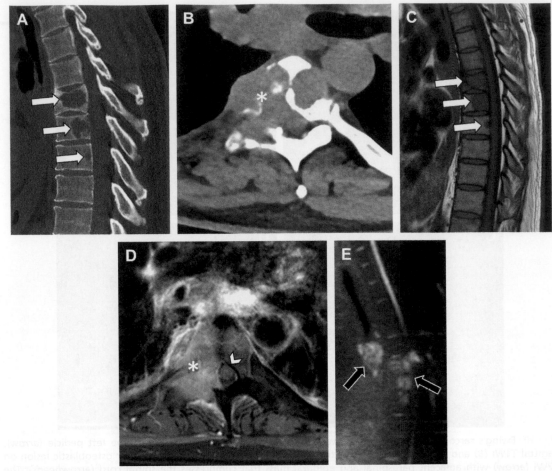

Fig. 12. Metastases. Sagittal (*A*) and axial (*B*) CT images show multiple osteolytic lesions involving various vertebral bodies (*arrows* in *A*). A right paraspinal soft tissue mass extends to the epidural space (*asterisk*). Sagittal T1WI (*C*) demonstrates multiple metastatic lesions involving several thoracic vertebral bodies (*white arrows*), and postcontrast axial T1WI (*D*) shows an epidural mass (*asterisk*) that displaces the spinal cord (*arrowhead*). The right paraspinal and the vertebral body lesions demonstrate restricted diffusion (*black arrows*) in sagittal diffusion weighted images (DWI) (*E*). Subcarinal nodes are seen on axial images.

improvement in quality of life and reduced complications.[39–41]

There are three types of bone metastases in the spine: around 71% are osteolytic, 8% osteoblastic, and 21% mixed. MR imaging is the preferred method for evaluating metastatic spine disease. Owing to the trabecular bone origin of these lesions, destruction of around 50% to 75% of the bone must be seen so that they can be visualized in radiography.[42,43] MR imaging gives a better characterization of the bone marrow lesions, soft tissue involvement, and epidural invasion. Metastatic bone compromise is usually seen as focal or multifocal lesions and less common as a diffuse compromise. T1WI plays an essential role in detecting diffuse compromise, and the disc and paraspinal musculature is used as a control in these cases. Diffuse marrow-replacing tumors appear hypointense to normal marrow on T1 and

isointense to hypointense to the vertebral disc or musculature. Focal metastases show hypointense signal on T1WI, in contrast with the T1 hyperintense normal surrounding bone marrow with high

Table 3 Most common location of extradural tumors	
Location	
Vertebral Body	*Neural Arch*
Enostosis	Osteoid Osteoma
Giant cell tumor	Osteoblastoma
Hemangioma	Aneurysmal bone cyst
Chordomas	Osteochondroma
Osteosarcoma	Osteosarcoma
Chondrosarcoma	Chondrosarcoma
Metastasis	Ewing sarcoma

Table 4
Location of extradural tumors found in distinct segments of vertebral spine

	Location
Cervical	Osteochondroma (C2) Osteoblastoma Aneurysmal bone cyst (40%) Hemangioma
Thoracic	Chondrosarcoma Osteoblastoma Osteosarcoma Hemangioma
Lumbar	Osteoid Osteoma Osteoblastoma Osteosarcoma Hemangioma
Sacrum	Giant cell tumor Chondrosarcoma Chordoma Ewing Sarcoma

fat percentage. Given the water content in lytic lesions, T2 and STIR images demonstrate hyperintense signal that can mix with the surrounding bone marrow edema. Osteoblastic and highly sclerotic lesions demonstrate low signal in T1WI and T2WI due to the lack of water. Using T1WI and STIR images alone has shown to be effective in diagnosing spinal metastases. Post-contrast images aid in the evaluation of extraosseous extension and in the assessment of leptomeningeal spread.[39,42] Spine metastases can be associated with pathologic fractures, which may be challenging to distinguish from benign compression fractures. Imaging features that suggest

malignancy include multifocal disease, involvement of the posterior wall or pedicles, and extension into the epidural and paraspinal spaces.[39] Owing to the high cellularity and low water content in metastases, DWI demonstrates low apparent diffusion coefficient (ADC) values and has shown to be effective as a complementary sequence, in evaluating treatment response and differentiating benign versus malignant fractures.[44]

SUMMARY

SE tumors are rare and often diagnosed incidentally. Primary tumors are usually benign; nonetheless, they can have aggressive behavior and cause significant morbidity and mortality due to proximity to multiple neural structures. Imaging plays an essential role in the detection and evaluation of complications. However, because imaging findings of SE tumors could overlap, age, location, and clinical presentation aid in correctly diagnosing and managing these neoplasms. Some of the characteristics that may aid in the diagnosis are summarized in Tables 3–5.

CLINICS CARE POINTS

- Primary bone tumors of the spine represent a wide variety of neoplasms that represent less than 5% of all bone tumors.

- Although imaging appearances are not always pathognomonic, the use of different imaging modalities assists the radiologist to narrow the differential diagnosis and determine the extension of the disease.

- Clinical presentation, location, size, and borders' appearance are important clues to make an imaging-based diagnosis.

Table 5
Prevalence of diagnosis of extradural tumors within age groups

	Age
<30	Osteoid Osteoma (10–20) Osteoblastoma (10–30) Aneurysmal bone cyst (<20) Giant cell tumor (20–40) Osteochondroma (20–40) Hemangioma Ewing sarcoma
30–50	Hemangioma Osteochondroma (20–40) Chordoma (40–60) Osteosarcoma Chondrosarcoma
>50	Hemangioma Chordoma (40–60) Osteosarcoma

DISCLOSURE

The authors have nothing to disclose.

REFERENCES

1. Murp D. Primary Tumors of the Spine. Radiologic-Pathologic Correlatio& 1996;16(5):28.
2. Vidal JA, Murphey MD. Primary Tumors of the Osseous Spine. Magn Reson Imag Clin N Am 2007;15(2):239–55.
3. Shah J, Gandhi D, Chauhan A, et al. Imaging Review of Pediatric Benign Osteocytic Tumors and Latest Updates on Management. J Clin Med 2021;10(13):2823.

4. Wald JT. Imaging of Spine Neoplasm. Radiol Clin North Am 2012;50(4):749–76.

5. Tepelenis K, Skandalakis GP, Papathanakos G, et al. Osteoid Osteoma: An Updated Review of Epidemiology, Pathogenesis, Clinical Presentation, Radiological Features, and Treatment Option. In Vivo 2021;35(4):1929–38.

6. Van Goethem JWM, van den Hauwe L, Özsarlak Ö, et al. Spinal tumors. Eur J Radiol 2004;50(2):159–76.

7. Kan P, Schmidt MH. Osteoid Osteoma and Osteoblastoma of the Spine. Neurosurg Clin N Am 2008; 19(1):65–70.

8. Rodallec MH, Feydy A, Larousserie F, et al. Diagnostic Imaging of Solitary Tumors of the Spine: What to Do and Say. Radiographics 2008;28(4): 1019–41.

9. Orguc S, Arkun R. Primary Tumors of the Spine. Semin Musculoskelet Radiol 2014;18(03):280–99.

10. Abdel Razek AAK, Castillo M. Imaging appearance of primary bony tumors and pseudo-tumors of the spine. J Neuroradiol 2010;37(1):37–50.

11. Luther N, Bilsky MH, Härtl R. Giant Cell Tumor of the Spine. Neurosurg Clin N Am 2008;19(1):49–55.

12. Tsukamoto S, Mavrogenis AF, Langevelde K van, et al. Imaging of Spinal Bone Tumors: Principles and Practice. Curr Med Imaging Former Curr Med Imaging Rev 2022;18(2):142–61.

13. Burch S, Hu S, Berven S. Aneurysmal Bone Cysts of the Spine. Neurosurg Clin N Am 2008;19(1):41–7.

14. Restrepo R, Zahrah D, Pelaez L, et al. Update on aneurysmal bone cyst: pathophysiology, histology, imaging and treatment. Pediatr Radiol 2022;52(9): 1601–14.

15. Mankin HJ, Hornicek FJ, Ortiz-Cruz E, et al. Aneurysmal Bone Cyst: A Review of 150 Patients. J Clin Oncol 2005;23(27):6756–62.

16. Carlos-Escalante JA, Paz-López ÁA, Cacho-Díaz B, et al. Primary Benign Tumors of the Spinal Canal. World Neurosurg 2022;164:178–98.

17. Anaya JEC, Coelho SRN, Taneja AK, et al. Differential Diagnosis of Facet Joint Disorders. Radiographics 2021;41(2):543–58.

18. Yang C, Zhang R, Lin H, et al. Insights into the molecular regulatory network of pathomechanisms in osteochondroma. J Cell Biochem 2019;120(10): 16362–9.

19. Fowler J, Takayanagi A, Fiani B, et al. Diagnosis, Management, and Treatment Options: A Cervical Spine Osteochondroma Meta-Analysis. World Neurosurg 2021;149:215–25.e6.

20. Peckham ME, Hutchins TA. Imaging of Vascular Disorders of the Spine. Radiol Clin North Am 2019; 57(2):307–18.

21. Leong S, Kok HK, Delaney H, et al. The Radiologic Diagnosis and Treatment of Typical and Atypical Bone Hemangiomas: Current Status. Can Assoc Radiol J 2016;67(1):2–11.

22. Riahi H, Mechri M, Barsaoui M, et al. Imaging of Benign Tumors of the Osseous Spine. J Belg Soc Radiol 2018;102(1):13.

23. Sekar A, Datta D, Parameshwar, et al. Aggressive vertebral hemangiomas in children. Childs Nerv Syst 2022;22. https://doi.org/10.1007/s00381-022-05760-9.

24. Murphey MD, Minn MJ, Contreras AL, et al. Imaging of spinal chordoma and benign notochordal cell tumor (BNCT) with radiologic pathologic correlation. Skeletal Radiol 2022;5. https://doi.org/10.1007/s00256-022-04158-7.

25. Sciubba DM, Chi JH, Rhines LD, et al. Chordoma of the Spinal Column. Neurosurg Clin N Am 2008; 19(1):5–15.

26. Pennington Z, Ehresman J, McCarthy EF, et al. Chordoma of the sacrum and mobile spine: a narrative review. Spine J 2021;21(3):500–17.

27. Tirabosco R, O'Donnell P, Flanagan AM. Notochordal Tumors. Surg Pathol Clin 2021;14(4): 619–43.

28. Wang VY, Potts M, Chou D. Sarcoma and the Spinal Column. Neurosurg Clin N Am 2008;19(1):71–80.

29. McLoughlin GS, Sciubba DM, Wolinsky JP. Chondroma/Chondrosarcoma of the Spine. Neurosurg Clin N Am 2008;19(1):57–63.

30. Moussalem CK, Massaad E, Baassiri W, et al. Spinal sarcomas and immunity: An undervalued relationship. Semin Cancer Biol 2020;64:36–50.

31. Pennington Z, Ehresman J, Pittman PD, et al. Chondrosarcoma of the spine: a narrative review. Spine J 2021;21(12):2078–96.

32. Kurugoglu S, Adaletli I, Mihmanli I, et al. Lumbosacral osseous tumors in children. Eur J Radiol 2008; 65(2):257–69.

33. Zamagni E, Cavo M. The role of imaging techniques in the management of multiple myeloma. Br J Haematol 2012;12007. https://doi.org/10.1111/bjh.

34. Ormond Filho AG, Carneiro BC, Pastore D, et al. Whole-Body Imaging of Multiple Myeloma: Diagnostic Criteria. Radiographics 2019;39(4):1077–97.

35. Lasocki A, Gaillard F, Harrison SJ. Multiple myeloma of the spine. NeuroRadiol J 2017;30(3):259–68.

36. Kosmala A, Bley T, Petritsch B. Bildgebende Diagnostik des Multiplen Myeloms. Tumordiagn Ther 2020;41(04):246–57.

37. Spratt DE, Beeler WH, de Moraes FY, et al. An integrated multidisciplinary algorithm for the management of spinal metastases: an International Spine Oncology Consortium report. Lancet Oncol 2017; 18(12):e720–30.

38. Hernandez RK, Adhia A, Wade SW, et al. Prevalence of bone metastases and bone-targeting agent use among solid tumor patients in the United States. Clin Epidemiol 2015;335. https://doi.org/10.2147/CLEP.S85496.

39. Jabehdar Maralani P, Lo SS, Redmond K, et al. Spinal metastases: multimodality imaging in diagnosis and stereotactic body radiation therapy planning. Future Oncol 2017;13(1):77–91.

40. Mossa-Basha M, Gerszten PC, Myrehaug S, et al. Spinal metastasis: diagnosis, management and follow-up. Br J Radiol 2019;92(1103):20190211.

41. Ong W, Zhu L, Zhang W, et al. Application of Artificial Intelligence Methods for Imaging of Spinal Metastasis. Cancers 2022;14(16):4025.

42. Pinter NK, Pfiffner TJ, Mechtler LL. Neuroimaging of spine tumors. Handb Clin Neurol 2016;136:689–706.

43. Donthineni R. Diagnosis and Staging of Spine Tumors. Orthop Clin North Am 2009;40(1):1–7.

44. Oztekin O, Ozan E, Hilal Adibelli Z, et al. SSH-EPI diffusion-weighted MR imaging of the spine with low b values: is it useful in differentiating malignant metastatic tumor infiltration from benign fracture edema? Skeletal Radiol 2009;38(7):651–8.

Diffusion Weighted Imaging in Spine Tumors

Sema Yildiz, MD[a],*, Michael Schecht, MD[a], Amit Aggarwal, MD[a], Kambiz Nael, MD[b], Amish Doshi, MD[a], Puneet S. Pawha, MD[a]

KEYWORDS

- Diffusion weighted imaging • Diffusion tensor imaging • ADC • FA • Multiple myeloma
- Malignant fracture • Intramedullary spinal cord tumor

KEY POINTS

- Advances in MR pulse-sequence design have resulted in significant improvement in the quality and increased utilization of spine diffusion weighted imaging (DWI) and diffusion tensor imaging (DTI) in recent years.
- DWI has developed into a valuable tool in evaluating vertebral body lesions, both for lesion detection and treatment response, particularly in multiple myeloma.
- As opposed to most regions of the body, both vertebral and spinal cord tumors tend to have higher apparent diffusion coefficient (ADC) values than their normal background tissues.
- DWI and ADC values may help in the differentiation between malignant and osteoporotic fractures, with lower ADC values in malignant infiltration.
- DTI fiber tractography can be used to characterize the relationship of a cord lesion with the adjacent spinal cord white matter tracts. The pattern of involvement can help distinguish between infiltrative and circumscribed tumors and can be valuable in surgical planning.

INTRODUCTION

Diffusion weighted imaging (DWI) is a powerful magnetic resonance (MR) imaging technique that can evaluate diffusion properties of physiologic tissues and provide insight about the microstructural construct. By sensitizing the MR acquisition to perturbations of the random motion of water molecules, DWI has become a valuable tool for tissue investigation, providing unique insight into pathogenesis of various disease states. Although the killer application has been in the assessment of brain disorders and cerebral ischemia, extracranial applications of DWI, particularly in the assessment of abdominal, breast, and prostate pathologic conditions, have increased exponentially in the last decade.[1–4]

Although DWI is a less widespread application in the spine, it has played an increasingly important role in the assessment of spinal tumors during recent years, particularly in the assessment of vertebral marrow lesions such as multiple myeloma and metastatic disease. Intramedullary cord tumors represent another arena where DWI, as well as diffusion tensor imaging (DTI) and fiber tractography, can play a valuable role in both diagnostic evaluation and surgical planning. This review discusses the current techniques and applications of DWI and DTI in the imaging evaluation of spine tumors.

DWI is less frequently used for the assessment of spine pathologic condition, when compared with the brain, in part due to inherent artifacts associated with this technique. However, during the years, advances in sequence design and MR imaging technology, including higher gradient MR systems and parallel imaging, have resulted in significant improvement in the quality of spine DWI.

The authors have no relevant disclosures.
[a] Division of Neuroradiology, Department of Radiology, Icahn School of Medicine at Mount Sinai Hospital, 1468 Madison Avenue MC Level, New York, NY 10029, USA; [b] Division of Neuroradiology, Department of Radiology, Ronald Reagan UCLA Medical Center, 757 Westwood Plaza, Los Angeles, CA 90095, USA
* Corresponding author.
E-mail address: Sema.Yildiz@mountsinai.org

Neuroimag Clin N Am 33 (2023) 459–475
https://doi.org/10.1016/j.nic.2023.04.001
1052-5149/23/Published by Elsevier Inc.

neuroimaging.theclinics.com

IMAGE ACQUISITION AND TECHNICAL CONSIDERATIONS

Since its introduction in the early 1990s,[5] DWI has been traditionally obtained by use of echo planar imaging (EPI). The main advantage of EPI is related to its fast acquisition time. However, EPI is prone to several artifacts including geometric distortions, image blurring, and ghosting artifacts[6,7] (Box 1). Alternative techniques based on single-shot and line scan fast spin echo,[8,9] with presumed advantages over EPI, have been investigated but failed to achieve broad clinical acceptance.

EPI diffusion weighted sequences are acquired at low and high b-values, which are used to calculate the apparent diffusion coefficient (ADC). High b-value images are acquired in at least 3 directions, which are averaged together to construct a set of trace DWI images, typically used for visual evaluation. Trace DWI images have both a diffusion component and T2 weighting contributing to signal, whereas ADC maps reflect only water diffusion.

With advances in pulse-sequence design and MR technology, different flavors of EPI-based DWI have been developed and evolved over time. The main technical consideration for EPI-based DWI for spine imaging is to minimize the time to echo (TE) in order to improve signal to noise ratio (SNR) and reduce the distortion. Below, we describe 3 commonly used EPI-based approaches for imaging of the spinal column, which include single shot EPI (ss-EPI), single-shot reduced field-of-view optimized and constrained undistorted single-shot (FOCUS)-EPI,[10] and readout-segmented EPI (rs-EPI),[11] with a brief discussion about incremental added value in diagnostic image quality (Table 1).

Single Shot Echo Planar Imaging

It is considered the entry level EPI technique for DWI imaging and is widely available on almost all MR scanners. However, its routine application without proper modifications can be challenging, due to significant distortions imposed by susceptibility variation associated with the osseous

> **Box 1**
> **Limitations and artifacts of spinal diffusion tensor imaging**
>
> - Susceptibility artifacts
> - Geometric distortion
> - Low SNR
> - Ghosting artifacts
> - Imaging blurring

structures and field variations adjacent to the spinal column (air in the lungs, blood vessels, abdominal viscera, and so forth).

Minor modifications can be made to current EPI-based parameters to increase diagnostic image quality. These include using lower B values (400–500) and limiting the number of phase encoding steps (usually to less than 128), both of which can result in minimizing TEs, which in turn can reduce distortion and increase SNR. Furthermore, introduction of multicoil technology for spine imaging and application of parallel imaging can further decrease the number of phase encodings and further decrease the TE.

Single Shot Reduced Field of View Echo Planar Imaging (FOCUS)

The major limitation of ss-EPI is related to its long readout duration, which can result in significant image artifacts including motion, ghosting, and distortion. FOCUS method was developed to reduce the required readout duration for ss-EPI, mitigating image artifact.[10] In this method, restricted field of view (FOV) is obtained by applying a 2D spatially selective echo-planar RF excitation pulse and a 180° refocusing pulse, to reduce the FOV in the phase-encoded direction. This reduced FOV method enables higher resolution for a fixed readout length and allows for contiguous multislice imaging without the need for interslice gaps (Fig. 1).

Readout-Segmented Echo Planar Imaging

In this technique, by applying phase-navigated multishot-interleaved technique, k-space is acquired in multiple interleafs (or lines).[11,12] By doing so, a more rapid acquisition through k-space (in the phase-encoding direction) is obtained, which in turn can result in the reduction of motion-related artifacts. There is also improvement in echo train length and susceptibility distortion. Incorporation of parallel imaging to this technique can further reduce acquisition time and reduce TE, which in turn can improve geometric distortion and blurring artifacts.[13,14]

Whole Body Diffusion Weighted Imaging

During the last decade, and with improvement in MR imaging technology, including availability of moving tables and multisurface receiver coil arrays, there has been an increasing interest in applying whole body diffusion weighted imaging (WB-DWI). The main applications have been in the detection and staging of a variety of oncological diseases, such as lymphoma or metastases.[15–18] One of the fastest growing applications

Table 1
Sample parameters for lumbar spine diffusion tensor imaging

	Single Shot EPI	Readout Segmented EPI	Restricted FOV EPI
TR/TE (ms)	4900/minimum	3000/56	4000/minimum
FOV (mm)	260 × 200	260 × 160	280 × 120
Matrix size (mm)	64 × 192	70 × 194	60 × 160
Slices (n) × thickness (mm)	16 × 4	15 × 3	16 × 4
Diff directions	6	3	3 in 1
B values (s/mm²)	0,1000 (*can switch to 400, same acq time*)	0,400	50 ,400
Parallel acquisition	2	2	2
Acquisition time (s)	86	137	228

of WB-DWI has been in patients with myeloma. WB-DWI has been shown to be a highly sensitive quantitative imaging technique for detecting diffuse and multifocal marrow infiltration, in patients with myeloma.[19] It can therefore be used not only for diagnosis and staging but also for treatment response assessment and outcome.[20]

VERTEBRAL BODY LESIONS

DWI has developed into an important tool for the evaluation of marrow replacing vertebral body lesions, allowing both qualitative and quantitative assessment. Normal adult bone marrow demonstrates relatively low ADC values. This is hypothesized to be a result of the high fat content in normal adult yellow marrow, which limits extracellular water content and restricts water motion, partly due to its hydrophobic nature.[21,22] Another contributing factor may be relatively lower blood flow and thus a lower perfusion component to

the ADC value, as compared with red marrow.[22] As a result, ADC decreases normally during maturation as red marrow is replaced by yellow marrow. Additionally, and in contradistinction to the soft tissues, malignant lesions of the spine generally demonstrate higher ADC values than normal fatty adult bone marrow. The typical ADC value of normal adult yellow marrow ranges between 0.2 and 0.5×10^{-3} mm²/s, whereas infiltrated marrow is typically between 0.7 and 1.0×10^{-3} mm²/s[22,23] (**Box 2**). This is somewhat counterintuitive as lesions are often described as "diffusion restricting." It should therefore be understood that this does not necessarily imply they have a lower ADC signal than the background or "normal" marrow. Given the variability in marrow composition, both in the course of normal growth and development, as well as in the posttreatment setting, interpretation of diffusion signal can be complex.

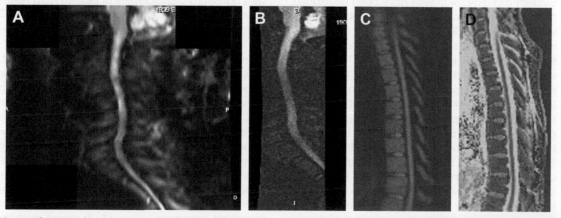

Fig. 1. Three EPI-based approaches for DWI of the spine. Single shot EPI (*A*) and single-shot reduced field-of-view FOCUS-EPI (*B*) performed on the same patient. Note the improvement in distortion when applying reduced FOV. Readout-segmented EPI (*C, D*) on a different patient, with trace and ADC maps. Note the high anatomic fidelity, and the absence of distortion and motion artifact.

> **Box 2**
> **Vertebral body diffusion imaging**
>
> - Normal adult yellow marrow tends to have a relatively lower ADC value compared with pathologic marrow
> - Degree of fat content and perfusion contribute to the observed ADC signal in bone marrow
> - ADC value of normal adult yellow marrow: $0.2–0.5 \times 10^{-3}$ mm^2/s
> - Pathologic marrow: $0.7–1.0 \times 10^{-3}$ mm^2/s

Multiple Myeloma

Lesion detection

Historically, the evaluation of multiple myeloma relied on radiographic spine survey studies. This is now being largely replaced by more modern and sensitive imaging modalities. Whole body MR (WB-MR) imaging, which includes DWI sequences, is now an important part of international guidelines for the imaging assessment of multiple myeloma.[24,25]

Five general MR imaging patterns of intramedullary myeloma have been described. These are focal disease, homogeneous diffuse disease, combined focal and diffuse disease, heterogenous salt and pepper pattern (or micronodular), and normal marrow.[24,26] Lesions may be identified by T1 hypointensity (compared with normal yellow bone marrow), hyperintensity on short tau invesion recovery (STIR) images, contrast enhancement, and diffusion hyperintensity (Fig. 2).

Recently, in the interest of standardization of diagnosis and treatment response evaluation, the Myeloma Response Assessment and Diagnosis System (MY-RADS) criteria have been developed, of which DWI is a critical part.[26] Generally, 2 b values (low, 50–100 s/mm^2; and high 800–900 s/mm^2) and calculated ADC maps are included with standard WB-MR imaging protocols. The lower b value maps have the benefit of higher SNR at the cost of sensitivity to perfusion effects and are therefore obtained primarily for ADC calculation.[22] Higher b value maps suppress more normal background signal, increasing sensitivity to diffusion hyperintense lesions but with relatively lower SNR.[27] In general, the high b value maps are used clinically for lesion detection. Focal lesions are defined as measuring at least 5 mm in size. Active lesions will demonstrate hyperintense signal on the high b value maps. However, hyperintensity due to nonneoplastic reasons, such as infection, fracture, or degenerative changes can result in false positives. Correlation with conventional sequences is essential. Additionally, ADC value measurement allows further differentiation. ADC values of active focal myelomatous lesions range between 0.7 and 1.4×10^{-3} mm^2/s, higher than normal background marrow, although less than fluid. Diffuse marrow involvement may be suspected when there is diffusely elevated signal on high b-value images. This may be confirmed with abnormal ADC values measured in a representative region of interest of approximately 1 cm^2.[26]

The importance of detection of focal lesions has prognostic implications because patients with focal lesions are found to have poorer outcomes. Early detection can therefore lead to alteration of treatment strategy.[26] In a study of 36 patients, increased detection of focal lesions with DWI led to clinical upstaging when compared with contrast-enhanced MR.[28] MR imaging with DWI has also been shown to be superior to other cross-sectional modalities. In one study of 49 patients, DWI showed greater sensitivity than fluorodeoxyglucose (FDG) positron emission tomogrophy/computed tomography (PET-CT) for detection of intramedullary lesions outside the skull. Detection of soft tissue extramedullary lesions was equivalent between these 2 modalities.[29]

Treatment response

Response assessment is based on the complex evolution of signal change within lesions after treatment. In treatment responders, there is an initial increase in ADC values in target lesions, as well as more diffusely in the skeleton.[25] This is suspected to reflect a decrease in tumor cellularity related to tumor cell necrosis, as well as a component of treatment-related edema. In a prospective study including 7 patients with myeloma and 8 healthy volunteers, this was demonstrated as a rightward displacement of plotted ADC histograms, indicating an overall increase in ADC signal. A 3.3% ADC increase was identified as being 90% sensitive and 100% specific for treatment response.[30] Nonresponders to treatment, however, showed no significant change in the appearance of the ADC histogram. Beginning 20 weeks after therapy, and following this initial phase of signal increase, there is an observed decrease in ADC values. This may represent the return of normal marrow content and increasing normal marrow fat.[27] MYRADS criteria incorporate these observed signal changes. ADC signal changes from 1.4×10^{-3} mm^2/s or lesser to $>1.4 \times 10^{-3}$ mm^2/s indicate high likelihood of treatment response[28] (Box 3). A recent systematic review of the literature and meta-analysis found a pooled sensitivity of 78% and specificity of 73% for DWI MR imaging in differentiating

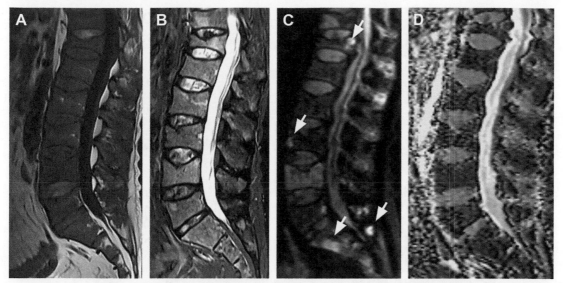

Fig. 2. Myeloma lesion detection with DWI. Lumbar spine MR images of a patient with multiple myeloma including T1, STIR, isotropic diffusion, and ADC sequences (*A–D*, respectively). There is increased conspicuity of a marrow replacing lesion involving the L4 vertebral body on the isotropic diffusion sequence (*C*) compared with the T1 and STIR images. Several smaller lesions are also more conspicuous, including S1 spinous process and multiple vertebral bodies (*arrows* in *C*).

treatment responders from nonresponders.[31] Interpretation of disease "activity" must consider the initial appearance of target lesions, as well as the timing since treatment (**Fig. 3**).

Intravoxel incoherent motion

Newer diffusion techniques are also being investigated for the evaluation of multiple myeloma. Among these is intravoxel incoherent motion (IVIM), which can evaluate perfusion effects on

---

Box 3
Diffusion imaging of multiple myeloma

- Several patterns of myeloma are observed on MR imaging. DWI is most important in detecting focal myelomatous lesions, which can change treatment and prognosis.

- Active hypercellular lesions will demonstrate hyperintense signal on the high b value maps with ADC values between 0.7 and 1.4×10^{-3} mm^2/s.

- After treatment, an initial increase in ADC values in lesions may reflect a decrease in tumor cellularity.

- 20 weeks after therapy, there is decrease in ADC values, which may represent the return of normal marrow content and increasing normal marrow fat.

- MYRADS criteria have been developed to standardize the radiologic assessment of myeloma diagnosis and treatment response.

ADC values. The diffuse pattern of myeloma has been shown to demonstrate significant increase in IVIM parameter D, the perfusion coefficient. Assessment of the vascularity of myeloma lesions with IVIM may also have utility in prognostication.[32]

Metastatic Disease

Lesion detection

DWI can also play a role in the detection and evaluation of metastatic vertebral body lesions. Metastatic lesions can also be highly cellular leading to diffusion restriction detectable on DWI (**Fig. 4**). Generally, osteolytic lesions are more readily detected on DWI imaging.[21] Sclerotic metastatic lesions will be less conspicuous on DWI due to the relative lack of water content.[23]

In a cohort of 36 patients with either breast or prostate cancer, DWI was found to provide increased sensitivity for lesion detection in patients with more than 10 lesions, when compared with bone scintigraphy.[33] DWI has also demonstrated superiority to 11C-methionine PET and bone scintigraphy in a subsequent study of 29 patients with bone metastases.[34] A more recent study of 39 patients with 239 total bony metastases demonstrated near equivalency of accuracy and sensitivity of osseous metastasis detection between whole body DWI MR imaging and FDG PET. The specificity was slightly lower, 87.8% versus 92.0%.[35]

Treatment response Recent literature has also addressed the role of DWI in the assessment of

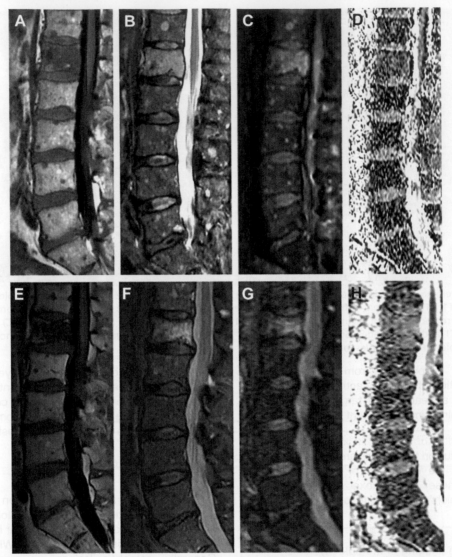

Fig. 3. Pretreatment and posttreatment imaging in multiple myeloma. T1, STIR, isotropic diffusion, and ADC map images from a patient with multiple myeloma before (*A–D*) and 4 months after (*E–H*) treatment. There is a dominant marrow replacing lesion at L1. After treatment, the lesion demonstrates mild increase in STIR signal (*F*). There is persistent diffusion hyperintense signal (*G*), with an increase in ADC signal (*H*). ADC value within an ROI of the L1 lesion measured 0.901×10^{-3} mm^2/s pretreatment, and 2.067×10^{-3} mm^2/s posttreatment. Interval development of mild pathologic compression fracture deformity of L1 is also identified.

treatment response.[36] One advantage of this technique is that it is not affected by posttreatment "flare" effects seen in bone scintigraphy. High b value and ADC signal measurements allow quantitative evaluation. Marked increases in ADC signal are generally indicative of favorable treatment response. Decrease, stability, or only modest increases of ADC signal are indicators of progression. However, the interplay of high b value, ADC, and morphologic signal can be complex.[37] In a recent pilot study of 21 patients with metastatic castration-resistant prostate cancer, decreases

in total lesional diffusion volume and increases in median ADC were shown to be indicators of treatment response[38] (**Box 4**).

Lymphoma

Whole body diffusion imaging has also been investigated as an alternative to PET-CT in staging and surveillance of patients with lymphoma. In general, DWI has been found to be equivalent to PET-CT in the evaluation of both nodal and extranodal involvement for staging purposes.[39] In one recent

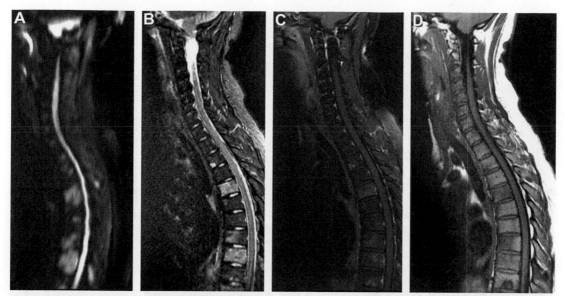

Fig. 4. Metastatic lesion detection with DWI. Isotropic diffusion (*A*), STIR (*B*), T1 postcontrast (*C*), and T1 precontrast (*D*) images from a patient with metastatic breast carcinoma. There are multiple marrow replacing lesions with high signal on the STIR sequence (*B*) and postcontrast enhancement (*C*) particularly in the T5, T8, and T9 vertebral bodies. These are also readily apparent on the diffusion sequence (*A*), which also shows 2 additional small spinous process lesions, not clearly seen in the other sequences.

study of 92 patients with lymphoma (both Hodgkins and non-Hodgkins), the diagnostic parameters of whole-body diffusion and PET-CT were compared with regard to nodal, solid organ, and bone marrow involvement. DWI outperformed PET-CT in bone marrow assessment, although was inferior in unenlarged nodal and splenic detection. Overall accuracy of staging was equivalent.[40]

Vertebral Fractures

Differentiation of benign osteoporotic vertebral body compression fractures from malignant pathologic fractures is a common clinical question. Diffusion imaging has also been investigated as a tool for this purpose (**Figs. 5** and **6**). The interplay of fracture age, underlying tumor cellularity, and

edema contribute to the signal changes on diffusion imaging in this setting.

In malignant compression fractures, the ADC will be comparatively lower, likely because of underlying malignant tumor cellularity. Edema and less-restricted water diffusion in osteoporotic fractures create higher ADC signal[27] (**Fig. 7**). However, both fracture types typically demonstrate a relatively higher ADC signal than surrounding normal bone marrow[23] (**Box 5**). In a study of 30 osteoporotic and 32 malignant compression fractures, axial DWI imaging was included to conventional protocols to assess the accuracy of diagnosis. Median ADC was found to be significantly lower in malignant fractures. Sensitivity, specificity, and accuracy all improved for differentiation of benign and malignant fractures, when conventional sequences with the addition of diffusion imaging was used, versus evaluation with conventional sequences only. The use of ADC ratios related to normal background marrow and adjacent paraspinal musculature also seem to aid in this evaluation.[41]

Other Primary Tumors

Primary malignant bone tumors are much less common than metastatic disease or myeloma. There are less data on the evaluation of untreated primary tumors compared with these other entities. Most of the literature focuses on lesions outside the vertebral column, particularly the

---

Box 4
Diffusion imaging of metastatic disease

- Metastatic lesions can show diffusion restriction due to high cellularity.
- Diffusion imaging is more useful for detecting lytic lesions but underperforms in the detection of sclerotic ones.
- Marked increases in ADC signal are generally indicative of favorable treatment response.
- Decrease, stability, or only modest increases of ADC signal are indicators of progression.

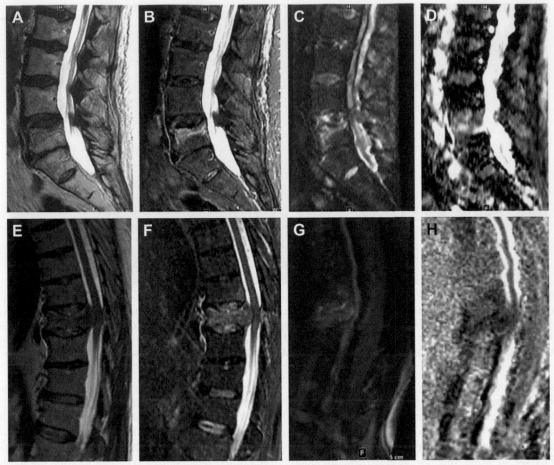

Fig. 5. Differentiation of benign and malignant compression fractures. T2, STIR, isotropic diffusion, and ADC maps from a patient with a benign osteoporotic compression fracture (*A–D*) and a separate patient with a malignant compression fracture (*E–H*). Aside from the epidural soft tissue component evident in the bottom row images, markedly low ADC signal can be seen in the malignant fracture (*H*), compared with the osteoporotic fracture (*D*).

extremities. One study found that DWI was helpful in discriminating between chondroblastic osteosarcomas and chondrosarcomas, with the former having significantly lower ADC signal than the latter.[42] This has important treatment and prognostic implications as surgery may be curative for chondrosarcomas, whereas chondroblastic osteosarcomas have a worse prognosis and require systemic therapy. More utility has been observed in the posttreatment setting. Increasing ADC values have been observed over multiple studies as being indicative of treatment response. In one study of 22 patients with osteosarcoma, minimum ADC value was determined to be a useful predictor of treatment response.[43] The ratio of pretreatment to posttreatment minimum and mean ADC values were calculated. Treatment responders had significantly higher posttreatment minimum ADC ratio compared with poor

response, although no difference was measured with mean ADC ratio value. Physiologic means of assessment can be especially useful because lesion size is not always decreased in the posttreatment setting, due to the residual mineralized tumor matrix.[44]

INTRAMEDULLARY SPINAL TUMORS AND TUMOR MIMICS

Long-term surgical outcome and surgical approach for spinal cord tumors is based on histological diagnosis and neurologic findings.[45–47] Total surgical resection of the tumor from the spinal cord is the goal for noninfiltrating intramedullary tumors, such as ependymoma and hemangioblastoma. Partial resection and subsequent radiotherapy are typically the approach for infiltrative tumors such as astrocytoma (grade 2 and higher).

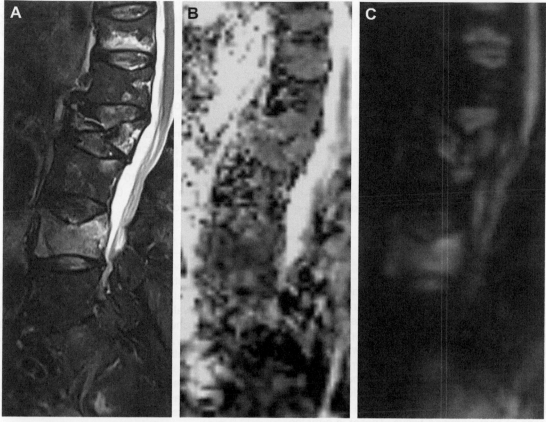

Fig. 6. Compression fractures in multiple myeloma. STIR, ADC map, and isotropic diffusion images (*A–C*, respectively) of a patient with multiple myeloma and multiple compression fractures. The background marrow signal measures 0.85×10^{-3} mm²/s. Severe compression deformity of L1 demonstrates an ADC value of 2.37×10^{-3} mm²/s and is likely osteoporotic or may represent treated disease. The active marrow replacing lesion at L3 with superimposed mild pathologic compression deformity, however, demonstrates a lower ADC value of 1.06×10^{-3} mm²/s.

Therefore, presurgical/pretreatment differentiation of infiltrating and noninfiltrating spinal cord tumors is essential. Conservative nonsurgical treatment strategy is appropriate for nonneoplastic tumor-like lesions such as tumefactive demyelination.

About 4% to 16% of suspected intramedullary tumors are found to be demyelinating lesions on histopathological evaluation.[48–50] Diffusion imaging can play a role in helping make these distinctions, in conjunction with conventional sequences.

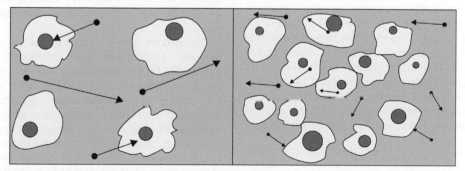

Fig. 7. Diffusion characteristics of benign and malignant fractures. In benign fractures, edema and increased extracellular space (*left panel*) results in facilitated diffusion, with corresponding higher ADC signal. In malignant fractures, increased cellularity results in relatively restricted movement of water molecules (*right panel*) and corresponding lower ADC signal, compared with benign fractures.

Diffusion Tensor Imaging of the Cord

DTI can play a valuable role in the evaluation of the spinal cord, particularly in assessing intramedullary tumors and their mimics. DTI allows quantitative and qualitative analysis of anisotropic diffusion, which refers to the directional bias of water diffusion based on tissue architecture and barriers. There is preferentially increased diffusion in the direction of intact white matter fibers, and relatively reduced diffusion perpendicular to the axon fibers, or in areas of compromised tissue. Tensor is a mathematical model, which is used to image this directional preference. There are at least 6 diffusion encoding directions (and often more than 20) assigned to each voxel: the diffusion coefficients along x, y, and z on the diagonal, and their covariances on the off-diagonal, which show correlation of random motions between each pair of principal direction. This matrix has 3 orthogonal eigenvectors for each voxel (I1, I2, and I3), which provides major and minor axes of the diffusion ellipsoid[51,52] (Fig. 8). Fractional anisotropy (FA) is the most widely used DTI-derived value and is defined as the root-mean-squared difference between each eigenvalue and the mean of the eigenvalues. The value of FA is scaled between 0 and 1. The directional anisotropic diffusion analysis is used to create three-dimensional fiber tractography, in which diffusion tensor streamlines provide graphical representation of spinal cord fiber tracts in craniocaudal and caudocranial orientation, allowing visual noninvasive assessment of spinal cord white matter tracts.

Apparent Diffusion Coefficient and Fractional Anisotropy Values of Cord Tumors

There have been several studies assessing FA and ADC values in intramedullary spinal cord tumors.[53–56] In one of the first case series, Ducreux

and colleagues[53] showed low FA values in intramedullary astrocytomas (FA 0.48 ± 0.02) compared with the spinal cord of healthy volunteers (FA 0.74 ± 0.04). Zhao and colleagues[55] also found significantly decreased FA (0.24 ± 0.11) and increased mean ADC values ([1.50 ± 0.52] × 10^{-3} mm^2/s) of cervical intramedullary astrocytomas when compared with healthy volunteers. Similar increased ADC findings were demonstrated in intramedullary pilocytic astrocytoma, a WHO I subtype tumor encountered in the pediatric population, with increased minimum ADC values of DWI (1.40 ± 0.28) × 10^{-3} mm^2/s, compared with (0.79 ± 0.05) × 10^{-3} mm^2/s in normal spinal cord.[57]

Tumor Versus Nonneoplastic Lesions

DWI with ADC values has a considerable value in making differential diagnosis of nontumoral intramedullary spinal cord lesions. Restricted diffusion with low ADC values is seen in acute demyelination, spinal cord ischemia, and intramedullary abscess. On the contrary, chronic spondylotic myelopathy, chronic demyelinating lesions, inflammatory lesions, and presyrinx state may show facilitated diffusion of water molecules with high ADC.[58]

Liu and colleagues[56] assessed the difference of FA values between intramedullary tumors (a combination of astrocytomas, ependymomas, and glioblastomas) and tumor-like lesions (multiple sclerosis, transverse myelitis, or sarcoidosis). They found reduced FA and increased ADC values in both tumor and tumor-like nonneoplastic lesions, compared with normal spinal cord. The nonneoplastic lesions demonstrated higher FA (0.39 vs 0.232) and lower ADC (0.862 × 10^{-3} mm^2/s vs 1.285 × 10^{-3} mm^2/s) values than the intramedullary tumors.[56] In a case report of autopsy-confirmed cervical spinal cord glioblastoma, premortally suspected to represent demyelinating disease on conventional MR imaging, decreased FA (0.293) was retrospectively noted within the lesion.[59]

Concordant with the findings of Liu and colleagues, Hohenhaus and colleagues[60] found decreased FA and increased mean ADC values at the tumor margins, and decreased FA values at the center of intramedullary tumors, when compared with inflammatory cord lesions. They included 18 intramedullary tumors: 10 ependymomas and 8 "other tumors" (7 glial tumors and one B-cell lymphoma). Mean FA at the margin of ependymomas was 0.322 (SD 0.147), 0.333 (SD 0.128) for other tumors, and 0.526 (SD 0.048) for inflammatory lesions. Mean FA values of ependymomas and other tumors at the lesion center was 0.240

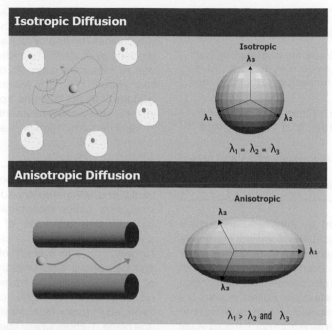

Fig. 8. Isotropic vs anisotropic diffusion. Upper image shows unrestricted diffusion with spherical distribution as seen in Cerebrospinal fluid (CSF), and to a lesser degree in gray matter. Lower image shows reduced diffusion perpendicular to white matter fiber tracts and preferential diffusion parallel to the tracts, resulting in an ellipsoid diffusion tensor.

(SD 0.099) and 0.249 (SD 0.106), respectively, whereas the FA of inflammatory lesions was 0.457 (SD 0.081). The mean ADC values were significantly higher at the lesion margin: 1.528 (SD 0.265) $\times$ 10^{-3} mm^2/s for ependymoma, 1.487 (SD 0.273) $\times$ 10^{-3} mm^2/s for other tumors, and 1.027 (SD 0.241) $\times$ 10^{-3} mm^2/s for inflammatory lesions. They concluded that an indeterminate tumor-like lesion with an FA greater than 0.4 or ADC $\approx$ 1.0 $\times$ 10^{-3} mm^2/s could be indicative of inflammatory rather than neoplastic disease and postulated this to reflect greater preservation of tissue integrity, resulting in less derangement of diffusion along fiber tracts in nontumoral entities.[60] Low FA values of tumoral lesions were thought to reflect disruption or displacement of parallel oriented highly anisotropic white matter fiber tracts.[56]

Tumor Infiltration Versus Edema

FA values can be useful in assessing peritumoral signal abnormality, potentially distinguishing peritumoral vasogenic edema from infiltrative tumor. Increased FA values were found in areas of signal change surrounding ependymomas, which are circumscribed tumors, compared with infiltrating astrocytic tumors at the peritumoral margins (0.399 (SD 0.08) vs 0.304 (SD 0.1)) and at the peritumoral edema (0.439 (SD 0.11) vs 0.350 (SD 0.1)), respectively.[60] This is presumably related to high cellularity of the peritumoral zone (both at the margin and at the edematous tissue) of infiltrating tumors[60] (Box 6).

Fiber Tractography Patterns of Cord Tumors

DTI fiber tractography can be used to visually evaluate the white matter tracts, represented by diffusion tensor streamlines, in relation to spinal cord tumors and nonneoplastic lesions.[54,61–66] Generally, fiber tracts can be either displaced, infiltrated/

Box 6
Diffusion tensor imaging and fractional anisotropy of spinal cord lesions

- Spinal cord tumors and many nonneoplastic cord lesions have lower FA and higher ADC values than normal spinal cord.

- Nonneoplastic lesions generally demonstrate higher FA and lower ADC values than intramedullary tumors.

- Low FA values of tumors reflect disruption or displacement of parallel oriented highly anisotropic white matter fibers.

- Infiltrative astrocytic tumors demonstrate lower peripheral FA compared with well-circumscribed ependymomas, due to higher tumor cellularity of the peritumoral zone.

encased, or disrupted by intramedullary tumors (Box 7). Well-circumscribed, noninfiltrating tumors smoothly displace tensor streamlines on fiber tractography. This is seen most commonly with ependymoma but can also be noted with hemangioblastoma and cord metastasis. Ependymomas are centrally located encapsulated tumors, known to have a good cleavage plane from normal cord. Axial FA maps will show a central defect, surrounded by preserved high FA at the periphery of the cord (Fig. 9). Smooth displacement or splaying of fibers can also be seen with grade I circumscribed astrocytomas, such as pilocytic astrocytomas in the pediatric population.[66] Moreover, in pediatric patients, tractography of lipomas can show a deformed and shifted conus medullaris, without destruction or disorganization of the fibers.[67]

In contradistinction, grade II and higher astrocytomas tend to infiltrate, encase, and/or disrupt diffusion tensor streamlines on tractography. Assessing the cystic components of astrocytomas is technically limited because tractography cannot properly evaluate the boundaries of a cystic tumor due to increased isotropic diffusivity of extracellular water[53] (Fig. 10). Moreover, Egger and colleagues[68] found that one spinal lymphoma case in their study showed an infiltrative pattern with streamline termination on tractography.

Tumor Resectability

Demonstration of the relationship between fiber tracts and intramedullary tumor can be used in evaluating tumor resectability, determination of surgical approach, use of neuronavigation for guiding the surgery, and clinical follow-up after surgery.[54,69,70] In a study of 14 patients, Setzer and colleagues[54] showed that the displacement of fibers with either no traversing fibers, or fibers crossing less than 50% of the lesion, corresponded to tumor resectability with a good cleavage plane. Tumors where fibers crossed more than 50% of the lesion or had complete infiltration/encasement of fibers, did not have a clear cleavage plane at surgery.[54]

Correlation between neurological examination and DTI fiber tractography findings has been shown.[71,72] No preoperative motor deficit was seen in cases where the cord tumor only displaced fiber tracts.[72] These findings were concordant with a study by Choudhri and colleagues,[66] evaluating DTI findings of pediatric intramedullary tumors. DTI fiber tractography-guided resection can

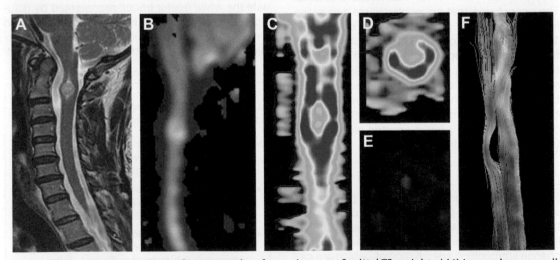

Fig. 9. Diffusion tensor imaging and tractography of ependymoma. Sagittal T2-weighted (*A*) image shows a well-defined, central intramedullary mass at the C2 level, without significant edema. The lesion is hyperintense on sagittal diffusion trace image (*B*). Coronal (*C*) and axial (*D*) FA maps, and axial color direction map (*E*), show preservation of peripherally displaced white matter tracts surrounding the central focal defect created by the intramedullary mass. Fiber tractography (*F*) demonstrates smooth outward displacement of white matter tracts surrounding the mass lesion, without infiltration.

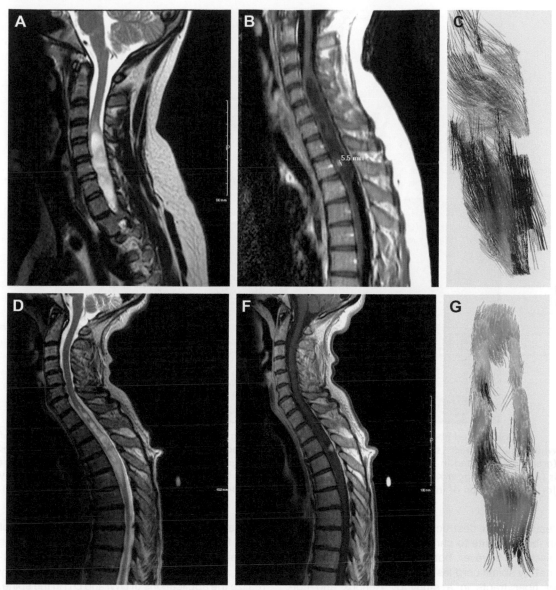

Fig. 10. Fiber tractography assessment of infiltrative vs well-circumscribed intramedullary tumors. A 17-year-old patient, with weakness and tingling in the right leg, is found to have an expansile heterogeneously T2 hyperintense (*A*) cervical cord lesion. The lesion is mostly nonenhancing, except for a subcentimeter enhancing nodule on sagittal T1 postcontrast image (*B*). Tractography (*C*) demonstrates an infiltrative pattern of diffusion tensor streamlines, and histopathologic evaluation confirmed the diagnosis of infiltrative astrocytoma. Sagittal T2 image (*D*) of a 69-year-old patient with right axillary pain and decreased proprioception shows long segment expansile T2 hyperintense signal involving the upper thoracic cord, including areas of syringomyelia. Sagittal T1 postcontrast (*E*) (*F*) shows a small enhancing dorsal spinal nodule at T3-T4 level. Tractography (*F*) (*G*) shows smooth displacement of the fiber tracts in this patient with hemangioblastoma. (*Courtesy of* C Torres, MD, FRCPC, FCAR, ON, Canada.)

facilitate adequate resection of the spinal cord tumor with preservation of neurologic function.[61,64]

Tractography of Tumor Mimics

Diffusion tractography findings can be helpful in differentiating acute demyelinating lesions from intramedullary tumors. Preserved normal pattern of fiber tracts can be seen traversing acute demyelinating lesions[68] (**Fig. 11**). In contrast, either displacement or disruption of fibers is noted in intramedullary tumors.[69] Gass and colleagues[73] argued that disruption of fibers can be noted, as a

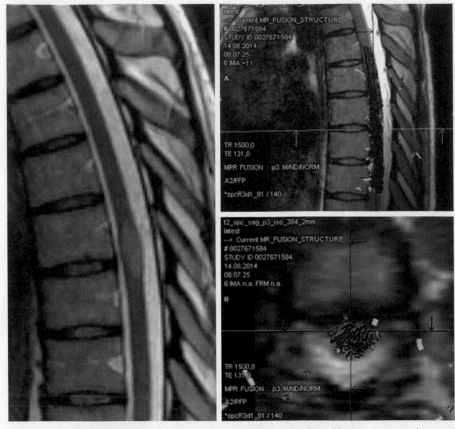

Fig. 11. Color-coded fiber tractography of an acute demyelinating spinal cord lesion. Preserved normal pattern of white matter tract streamlines is seen on direction-coded sagittal and axial tractography images (*green* = orientated in x-axis, *red* = y-axis, *blue* = z-axis). No significant disruption/infiltration or displacement is noted. (*From* Egger K, Hohenhaus M, Van Velthoven V, Heil S, Urbach H. Spinal diffusion tensor tractography for differentiation of intramedullary tumor-suspected lesions. Eur J Radiol. 2016;85(12):2275-2280.)

result of tissue destruction and axonal volume loss, in the subacute to chronic stage of demyelinating disease. However, both acute and chronic inflammatory spinal cord lesions showed only spreading of fiber tracts in a study by Renoux and colleagues,[74] suggesting edema without significant fiber disruption. Absence of substantial deviation or disruption of fibers has also been described in a case of radiation necrosis, which can mimic spinal tumors on conventional imaging.[75]

SUMMARY

DWI has grown into a powerful adjunctive tool in the evaluation of spine tumors, particularly for vertebral marrow lesions and intramedullary tumors. Advances in MR techniques have improved the quality of spine DWI and DTI in recent years, with increased reproducibility and utilization. DWI is now a component of the standardized criteria for the diagnosis and therapeutic assessment of multiple myeloma. DTI, with quantitative parameters

such as FA and qualitative visual assessment of nerve fiber tracts, can play a valuable role in the evaluation and surgical planning of spinal cord tumors. Although more studies are needed to fully realize the applications of DWI and DTI in the spine, these can currently be used with widely available techniques, to enhance the diagnostic and post-treatment evaluation of spinal tumors.

CLINICS CARE POINTS

- DWI is a valuable component of the standardized criteria for the diagnosis and therapeutic assessment of multiple myeloma.

- DWI plays a less formalized role in evaluating vertebral metastatic disease. It is more useful in detecting lytic rather than sclerotic lesions.

- DWI and ADC values may be helpful to differentiate benign osteoporotic fractures from malignant pathologic fractures, which is a common clinical question.

- DTI, with quantitative parameters like FA and qualitative visual assessment of nerve fiber tracts, can play a valuable role in the evaluation and surgical planning of spinal cord tumors.

REFERENCES

1. Taouli B, Koh DM. Diffusion-weighted MR imaging of the liver. Radiology 2010;254(1):47–66.
2. Barral M, Taouli B, Guiu B, et al. Diffusion-weighted MR imaging of the pancreas: current status and recommendations. Radiology 2015;274(1):45–63.
3. Thoeny HC, De Keyzer F. Extracranial applications of diffusion-weighted magnetic resonance imaging. Eur Radiol 2007;17(6):1385–93.
4. Lima M, Honda M, Sigmund EE, et al. Diffusion MRI of the breast: current status and future directions. J Magn Reson Imag 2020;52(1):70–90.
5. Le Bihan D. Molecular diffusion nuclear magnetic resonance imaging. Magn Reson Q 1991;7(1):1–30. PMID: 2043461.
6. Porter DA, Calamante F, Gadian DG, et al. The effect of residual Nyquist ghost in quantitative echo-planar diffusion imaging. Magn Reson Med 1999;42(2):385–92.
7. Stadlbauer A, Bernt R, Gruber S, et al. Diffusion-weighted MR imaging with background body signal suppression (DWIBS) for the diagnosis of malignant and benign breast lesions. Eur Radiol 2009;19(10):2349–56.
8. Gudbjartsson H, Maier SE, Mulkern RV, et al. Line scan diffusion imaging. Magn Reson Med 1996;36(4):509–19.
9. Xu D, Henry RG, Mukherjee P, et al. Single-shot fast spin-echo diffusion tensor imaging of the brain and spine with head and phased array coils at 1.5 T and 3.0 T. Magn Reson Imaging 2004;22(6):751–9.
10. Saritas EU, Cunningham CH, Lee JH, et al. DWI of the spinal cord with reduced FOV single-shot EPI. Magn Reson Med 2008;60(2):468–73.
11. Porter DA, Heidemann RM. High resolution diffusion-weighted imaging using readout-segmented echo-planar imaging, parallel imaging and a two-dimensional navigator-based reacquisition. Magn Reson Med 2009;62(2):468–75.
12. Bammer R, Augustin M, Prokesch RW, et al. Diffusion-weighted imaging of the spinal cord: interleaved echo-planar imaging is superior to fast spin-echo. J Magn Reson Imag 2002;15(4):364–73.
13. Holdsworth SJ, Skare S, Newbould RD, et al. Robust GRAPPA-accelerated diffusion-weighted readout-segmented (RS)-EPI. Magn Reson Med 2009; 62(6):1629–40.
14. Holdsworth SJ, Skare S, Newbould RD, et al. Readout-segmented EPI for rapid high resolution diffusion imaging at 3 T. Eur J Radiol 2008;65(1):36–46.
15. Lin C, Itti E, Luciani A, et al. Whole-body diffusion-weighted imaging with apparent diffusion coefficient mapping for treatment response assessment in patients with diffuse large B-cell lymphoma: pilot study. Invest Radiol 2011;46(5):341–9.
16. Laurent V, Trausch G, Bruot O, et al. Comparative study of two whole-body imaging techniques in the case of melanoma metastases: advantages of multi-contrast MRI examination including a diffusion-weighted sequence in comparison with PET-CT. Eur J Radiol 2010;75(3):376–83.
17. Kwee TC, Takahara T, Vermoolen MA, et al. Whole-body diffusion-weighted imaging for staging malignant lymphoma in children. Pediatr Radiol 2010; 40(10):1592–602 [quiz: 1720-1].
18. Gutzeit A, Doert A, Froehlich JM, et al. Comparison of diffusion-weighted whole body MRI and skeletal scintigraphy for the detection of bone metastases in patients with prostate or breast carcinoma. Skeletal Radiol 2010;39(6):333–43.
19. Pawlyn C, Fowkes L, Otero S, et al. Whole-body diffusion-weighted MRI: a new gold standard for assessing disease burden in patients with multiple myeloma? Leukemia 2016;30:1446–8.
20. Mai EK, Hielscher T, Kloth JK, et al. A magnetic resonance imaging-based prognostic scoring system to predict outcome in transplant-eligible patients with multiple myeloma. Haematologica 2015;100(6):818–25.
21. Filograna L, Magarelli N, Cellini F, et al. Diffusion weighted imaging (DWI) and apparent diffusion coefficient (ADC) values for detection of malignant vertebral bone marrow lesions. Eur Rev Med Pharmacol Sci 2018;22(3):590–7.
22. Subhawong TK, Jacobs MA, Fayad LM. Diffusion-weighted MR imaging for characterizing musculoskeletal lesions. Radiographics 2014;34(5):1163–77.
23. Dietrich O, Geith T, Reiser MF, et al. Diffusion imaging of the vertebral bone marrow. NMR Biomed 2015;30(3). https://doi.org/10.1002/nbm.3333.
24. Baffour FI, Glazebrook KN, Kumar SK, et al. Role of imaging in multiple myeloma. Am J Hematol 2020, 95(8):966–77.
25. Lecouvet FE, Vekemans M-C, Van Den Berghe T, et al. Imaging of treatment response and minimal residual disease in multiple myeloma: State of the art WB-MRI and PET/CT. Skeletal Radiol 2021;51(1):59–80.
26. Messiou C, Hillengass J, Delorme S, et al. Guidelines for Acquisition, interpretation, and reporting of whole-body MRI in myeloma: myeloma response assessment and diagnosis system (MY-RADS). Radiology 2019;291(1):5–13.

27. Van Den Berghe T, Verstraete KL, Lecouvet FE, et al. Review of diffusion-weighted imaging and dynamic contrast–enhanced MRI for multiple myeloma and its precursors (monoclonal gammopathy of undetermined significance and smouldering myeloma). Skeletal Radiol 2021;51(1):101–22.

28. Squillaci E, Bolacchi F, Altobelli S, et al. Pre-treatment staging of multiple myeloma patients: comparison of whole-body diffusion weighted imaging with whole-body T1-weighted contrast-enhanced imaging. Acta Radiologica 2015;56(6):733–8.

29. Chen J, Li C, Tian Y, et al. Comparison of whole-body DWI and 18F-FDG PET/CT for detecting intramedullary and extramedullary lesions in multiple myeloma. Am J Roentgenol 2019;213(3):514–23.

30. Giles SL, Messiou C, Collins DJ, et al. Whole-body diffusion-weighted MR imaging for assessment of treatment response in myeloma. Radiology 2014;271(3):785–94.

31. Torkian P, Mansoori B, Hillengass J, et al. Diffusion-weighted imaging (DWI) in diagnosis, staging, and treatment response assessment of multiple myeloma: a systematic review and meta-analysis. Skeletal Radiol 2023;52(3):565–83.

32. Torkian P, Azadbakht J, Andrea Bonaffini P, et al. Advanced imaging in multiple myeloma: new frontiers for MRI. Diagnostics 2022;12(9):2182.

33. Gutzeit A, Doert A, Froehlich JM, et al. Comparison of diffusion-weighted whole body MRI and skeletal scintigraphy for the detection of bone metastases in patients with prostate or breast carcinoma. Skeletal Radiol 2009;39(4):333–43.

34. Goudarzi B, Kishimoto R, Komatsu S, et al. Detection of bone metastases using diffusion weighted magnetic resonance imaging: comparison with 11C-methionine pet and Bone Scintigraphy. Magn Reson Imag 2010;28(3):372–9.

35. Sun W, Li M, Gu Y, et al. Diagnostic value of whole-body DWIi with background body suppression plus calculation of apparent diffusion coefficient at 3T versus 18F-FDG PET/CT for detection of bone metastases. Am J Roentgenol 2020;214(2):446–54.

36. Orcajo-Rincon J, Muñoz-Langa J, Sepúlveda-Sánchez JM, et al. Review of imaging techniques for evaluating morphological and functional responses to the treatment of bone metastases in prostate and breast cancer. Clin Transl Oncol 2022;24(7):1290–310.

37. Padhani AR, Makris A, Gall P, et al. Therapy monitoring of skeletal metastases with whole-body diffusion MRI. J Magn Reson Imag 2014;39(5):1049–78.

38. Perez-Lopez R, Mateo J, Mossop H, et al. Diffusion-weighted imaging as a treatment response biomarker for evaluating bone metastases in prostate cancer: a pilot study. Radiology 2017;283(1):168–77.

39. Stecco A, Buemi F, Lannessi A, et al. Current concepts in tumor imaging with whole-body MRI with diffusion imaging (WB-MRI-DWI) in multiple myeloma and lymphoma. Leuk Lymphoma 2018;59(11):2546–56.

40. Kharuzhyk S, Zhavrid E, Dziuban A, et al. Comparison of whole-body MRI with diffusion-weighted imaging and PET/CT in lymphoma staging. Eur Radiol 2020;30(7):3915–23.

41. Sung JK, Jee W-H, Jung J-Y, et al. Differentiation of acute osteoporotic and malignant compression fractures of the spine: Use of additive qualitative and quantitative axial diffusion-weighted MR imaging to conventional MR imaging at 3.0 T. Radiology 2014;271(2):488–98.

42. Yakushiji T, Oka K, Sato H, et al. Characterization of chondroblastic osteosarcoma: gadolinium-enhanced versus diffusion-weighted Mr Imaging. J Magn Reson Imag 2009;29(4):895–900.

43. Oka K, Yakushiji T, Sato H, et al. The value of diffusion-weighted imaging for monitoring the chemotherapeutic response of osteosarcoma: a comparison between average apparent diffusion coefficient and minimum apparent diffusion coefficient. Skeletal Radiol 2009;39(2):141–6.

44. Yao K, Troupis JM. Diffusion-weighted imaging and the skeletal system: a literature review. Clin Radiol 2016;71(11):1071–82.

45. Samartzis D, Gillis CC, Shih P, et al. Intramedullary spinal cord tumors: part I-epidemiology, pathophysiology, and diagnosis. Glob Spine J 2015;5(5):425–35.

46. Nakamura M, Ishii K, Watanabe K, et al. Surgical treatment of intramedullary spinal cord tumors: prognosis and complications. Spinal Cord 2008;46(4):282–6.

47. Jaiswal M, Shyam Mittal R. Outcome of operative intervention in intramedullary spinal cord tumors. Rom Neurosurg 2014;21:283–91.

48. Lee M, Epstein FJ, Rezai AR, et al. Nonneoplastic intramedullary spinal cord lesions mimicking tumors. Neurosurgery 1998;43(4):788–94 [discussion: 794-5].

49. Selviaridis P, Zountsas B, Chatzisotiriou A, et al. Demyelinating plaque imitates an intramedullary tumour. Clin Neurol Neurosurg 2007;109(10):905–9.

50. Wang Y, Wang M, Liang H, et al. Imaging and clinical properties of inflammatory demyelinating pseudotumor in the spinal cord. Neural Regen Res 2013;8(26):2484–94.

51. Basser PJ, Mattiello J, LeBihan D. MR diffusion tensor spectroscopy and imaging. Biophys J 1994;66(1):259–67.

52. Jellison BJ, Field AS, Medow J, et al. Diffusion tensor imaging of cerebral white matter: a pictorial review of physics, fiber tract anatomy, and tumor imaging patterns. AJNR Am J Neuroradiol 2004;25(3):356–69.

53. Ducreux D, Lepeintre JF, Fillard P, et al. MR diffusion tensor imaging and fiber tracking in 5 spinal cord astrocytomas. AJNR Am J Neuroradiol 2006;27(1): 214–6.

54. Setzer M, Murtagh RD, Murtagh FR, et al. Diffusion tensor imaging tractography in patients with intramedullary tumors: comparison with intraoperative findings and value for prediction of tumor resectability. J Neurosurg Spine 2010;13(3):371–80.

55. Zhao M, Shi B, Chen T, et al. Axial MR diffusion tensor imaging and tractography in clinical diagnosed and pathology confirmed cervical spinal cord astrocytoma. J Neurol Sci 2017;375:43–51.

56. Liu X, Tian W, Kolar B, et al. Advanced MR diffusion tensor imaging and perfusion weighted imaging of intramedullary tumors and tumor like lesions in the cervicomedullary junction region and the cervical spinal cord. J Neuro Oncol 2014;116(3):559–66.

57. She DJ, Lu YP, Xiong J, et al. MR imaging features of spinal pilocytic astrocytoma. BMC Med Imaging 2019;19(1):5.

58. Kim J, Bui DQ, Moritani T, et al. Spinal cord lesions. In: Moritani T, Capizzano AA, editors. Diffusion-weighted MR imaging of the brain, head and neck, and spine. Cham (Switzerland): Springer; 2021.

59. Liu X, Germin BI, Ekholm S. A case of cervical spinal cord glioblastoma diagnosed with MR diffusion tensor and perfusion imaging. J Neuroimaging 2011;21(3):292–6.

60. Hohenhaus M, Merz Y, Klingler JH, et al. Diffusion tensor imaging in unclear intramedullary tumor-suspected lesions allows separating tumors from inflammation. Spinal Cord 2022;60(7):655–63.

61. Mechtler LL, Nandigam K. Spinal cord tumors: new views and future directions. Neurol Clin 2013;31(1): 241–68.

62. Bloomer CW, Ackerman A, Bhatia RG. Imaging for spine tumors and new applications. Top Magn Reson Imaging 2006;17(2):69–87.

63. Baruah D, Chandra T, Bajaj M, et al. A simplified algorithm for diagnosis of spinal cord lesions. Curr Probl Diagn Radiol 2015;44(3):256–66.

64. Landi A, Palmarini V, D'Elia A, et al. Magnetic resonance diffusion tensor imaging and fiber-tracking diffusion tensor tractography in the management of spinal astrocytomas. World J Clin Cases 2016; 16(1):1–4, 4.

65. Alkherayf F, Arab AF, Tsai E. Conus Medullaris Teratoma with Utilization of Fiber Tractography: case Report. J Neurol Surg Rep 2015;76(1):e183–7.

66. Choudhri AF, Whitehead MT, Klimo P Jr, et al. Diffusion tensor imaging to guide surgical planning in intramedullary spinal cord tumors in children. Neuroradiology 2014;56(2):169–74.

67. Antherieu P, Levy R, De Saint Denis T, et al. Diffusion tensor imaging (DTI) and Tractography of the spinal cord in pediatric population with spinal lipomas: preliminary study. Childs Nerv Syst 2019;35(1):129–37.

68. Egger K, Hohenhaus M, Van Velthoven V, et al. Spinal diffusion tensor tractography for differentiation of intramedullary tumor-suspected lesions. Eur J Radiol 2016;85(12):2275–80.

69. Benjamin CG, Frempong-Boadu A, Hoch M, et al. Combined use of diffusion tractography and advanced intraoperative imaging for resection of cervical intramedullary spinal cord neoplasms: a case series and technical note. Oper Neurosurg (Hagerstown) 2019;17(5):525–30.

70. Granata F, Racchiusa S, Mormina E, et al. Presurgical role of MRI tractography in a case of extensive cervicothoracic spinal ependymoma. Surg Neurol Int 2017;8:56.

71. Phillips NS, Sanford RA, Helton KJ, et al. Diffusion tensor imaging of intraaxial tumors at the cervicomedullary and pontomedullary junctions. Report of two cases. J Neurosurg 2005;103(6 Suppl):557–62.

72. Czernicki T, Maj E, Podgórska A, et al. Diffusion tensor tractography of pyramidal tracts in patients with brainstem and intramedullary spinal cord tumors: Relationship with motor deficits and intraoperative MEP changes. J Magn Reson Imag 2017; 46(3):715–23.

73. Gass A, Rocca MA, Agosta F, et al, MAGNIMS Study Group. MRI monitoring of pathological changes in the spinal cord in patients with multiple sclerosis. Lancet Neurol 2015;14(4):443–54.

74. Renoux J, Facon D, Fillard P, et al. MR diffusion tensor imaging and fiber tracking in inflammatory diseases of the spinal cord. AJNR Am J Neuroradiol 2006;27(9):1947–51.

75. Keřkovský M, Zitterbartová J, Pour L, et al. Diffusion tensor imaging in Radiation-Induced Myelopathy. J Neuroimaging 2015;25(5):836–40.

Dynamic Contrast-Enhanced MR Perfusion
Role in Diagnosis and Treatment Follow-Up in Patients with Vertebral Body Tumors

Atin Saha, MD, MS[a,b,*], Kyung K. Peck, PhD[a], Sasan Karimi, MD[a,b],
Eric Lis, MD[b], Andrei I. Holodny, MD[a]

KEYWORDS

- DCE-MRI • Spine Metastases • Spine Treatment Response • Spine Perfusion

KEY POINTS

- Spinal metastases demonstrate elevated Vp and Ktrans on dynamic contrast-enhanced-MR imaging suggestive of viable tumor.
- Decreased quantitative perfusion parameters is suggestive of treatment response and nonviable disease.
- Vertebral body compression deformities with elevated Vp are likely pathologic in nature.
- Perfusion imaging of the spine can aid in discriminating hyper and hypovascular metastatic spine neoplasms as well as malignant and benign tumors.

INTRODUCTION

The diagnosis of cancer used to be synonymous with mortality. However, with the advent of new therapies and treatment approaches, many cancers have become a "chronic disease," allowing for longer survival times, even in patients with metastatic disease.[1] The key to improved survival is early diagnosis and subsequent treatment of cancer with keen eye toward early detection of treatment failure.

Treatment of metastatic disease is often similar to, or more challenging, than treating the isolated primary disease itself. When treating patients with cancer, it is essential to identify spinal metastases and gauge their response to treatment, as they can be found in up to 70% of patients with cancer.[2] Typically, conventional imaging techniques such as MR imaging, computed tomography (CT), PET, and bone scintigraphy have been used individually and in conjunction, to evaluate the presence of spinal metastases, extent of disease and treatment response. Using these techniques, assessing for viable tumor and therapy response can be at times challenging; more specifically, structural changes and imaging characteristics may not differ pretreatment and posttreatment on CT or MR imaging. However, advanced imaging techniques, such as dynamic contrast-enhanced (DCE) perfusion MR imaging, have been developed and show promise in improving and allowing for earlier detection of viable disease. This innovative technique is increasingly used for brain oncological imaging; however, this review focuses on its utility in the assessment of viable metastatic spinal disease. The authors discusses how DCE MR imaging can be used at various points in a patient's course of spine care to improve clinical outcomes.

DYNAMIC CONTRAST-ENHANCED-MR IMAGING
Background

Spinal tumor imaging with DCE-MR imaging is a relatively new perfusion MR imaging technique.[3]

[a] Department of Radiology, Memorial Sloan Kettering Cancer Center, 1275 York Avenue, New York, NY 10065, USA; [b] Department of Radiology, Weill Cornell Medical College, 1300 York Avenue, New York, NY 10065, USA
* Corresponding author.
E-mail address: sahaa@mskcc.org
Twitter: @AtinSaha (A.S.); @AndreiHolodny (A.I.H.)

Neuroimag Clin N Am 33 (2023) 477–486
https://doi.org/10.1016/j.nic.2023.03.006
1052-5149/23/© 2023 Elsevier Inc. All rights reserved.

The quantitative evaluation of the tumor microvasculature that DCE-MR imaging offers makes this method extremely useful in evaluating spinal metastases. Proangiogenic growth factors are released by spinal metastases,[4] which contributes to abnormal neo-angiogenesis with increased permeable vasculature, which can be characterized by DCE-MR imaging. The changes in tumor microenvironment occur before structural changes are appreciated on conventional MR imaging, thus DCE-MR imaging can capture these early changes and aid in identification of viable disease. Through quantitative parameters such as plasma volume (Vp), which is related to the number of blood vessels in the tumor, and the permeability constant (Ktrans), which is a measure of vasculature leakiness,[3] as well as using semiquantitative parameters such as area under the curve (AUC) of contrast uptake, DCE-MR imaging technique can noninvasively evaluate the vascular microenvironment and the hemodynamics of spinal neoplasms. DCE-MR imaging is a well-established imaging technique for the assessment of viable intracranial neoplasms[5,6] and has started to be used for the diagnosis and treatment monitoring of patients with spinal metastasis.[7,8]

Two-Compartment Model

DCE-MR imaging requires the dynamic, intravenous administration of gadolinium-based contrast agent, during which the patient is imaged periodically for several minutes before, during and after the contrast agent accumulates in the region of interest (ROI). The dynamic information acquired allows for characterization of tissue perfusion and vascular permeability. The data can be analyzed using quantitative and semiquantitative methods.

The extended pharmacokinetic two-compartment model developed by Tofts and colleagues, which uses voxel-wise tracer kinetic analysis, is the most widely selected quantitative method to analyze DCE data. This parametric method can fit a mathematical pharmacokinetic model to dynamically acquired tissue contrast concentration curves, so that quantitative tissue parameters (eg, permeability (Ktrans) and fractional plasma volume (Vp) that are related to vascularity) can be estimated. The two compartments include (1) extracellular extravascular space (EES) and (2) intravascular space (blood plasma).[9] Measured signal intensity changes over time are used for pharmacokinetic modeling of contrast agent uptake (Fig. 1). For an ROI, Vp estimates vascularity within the intravascular space, whereas Ktrans estimates vessel permeability by assessing volume transfer of contrast over time from the intravascular space to EES.

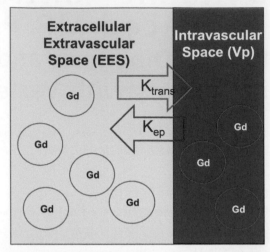

Fig. 1. A schematic illustration of pharmacokinetic two-compartment model. Tissue is presented as two compartments: the intravascular space (Vp) and extracellular extravascular space (EES). Gd, Gadolinium; Ktrans and Kep, volume transfer constants between Vp and EES.

Quantitative analysis relies on the detection of the arterial input function (AIF) from a large artery (typically the aorta for spine perfusion) within the imaging volume. Obtaining the AIF is needed to estimate the expected blood flow characteristics in the area of interest. The pixels that exhibit a large change in signal intensity, a quick shift immediately status post-bolus injection, and an early peak intensity are typically selected to confirm the appropriate shape of the AIF curve. Certain software packages have methods to automatically identify arteries to be used for the AIF curve.

Semiquantitative analysis is performed, via analyzing the averaged time-intensity curves (TICs) of changing MR signal intensity, during contrast accumulation for an ROI. Three parameters are extracted from TIC and include (1) peak enhancement signal percentage change ([signalmax −signalbase]/signalbase × 100%), (2) wash-in enhancement slope ([signalmax − signalbase]/timerise), and (3) AUC.[10,11]

Semiquantitative analysis has several advantages; it does not require the measurement of the AIF and several parameters such as AUC are relatively independent of contrast injection protocols.[12] However, one disadvantage is the fact that semiquantitative parameters do not correspond to definitive physiologic correlates. As they represent a combination of microcirculatory and tissue properties, the degree to which each of these physiologic parameters contributes to the contrast concentration curve remains unknown.[13] In addition, model-free methods remain sensitive to variations between different acquisition protocols, including scanner hardware stability, sequence parameters, scan duration, and amount of administered contrast.[13] Five types of TIC patterns have been described, Type A (nearly flat), Type B (slow rise in contrast enhancement), Type C (rapid wash-in followed by plateau), Type D (rapid wash-in then wash-out), and Type E (rapid wash-in followed by a second slow rise in contrast enhancement).[11]

Spine MR Imaging Acquisition: Protocol

The most widely used method of DCE-MR imaging data acquisition is 3D T1-weighted spoiled gradient-recalled echo. There is a newer 3D acquisition technique, known as differential subsampling with Cartesian ordering, which has demonstrated the ability to preserve spatial resolution while maintaining an effective temporal resolution of 3 to 4 seconds to characterize the kinetics of the contrast entry and exit out of the tissue.[14] To model the contrast concentration-TIC, post-contrast 3D T1-weighted images are acquired every 4 to 5 seconds, and in order to measure the signal shift caused by contrast injection, low flip angles (15°–25°) can be used. Short echo time can remove T2* effect of contrast and short repetition time can improve scan time.

CLINICAL APPLICATIONS
Discriminating Healthy Bone Marrow from Bone Metastases

Several studies have demonstrated extremely encouraging outcomes for the diagnosis of spinal metastases using DCE-MR imaging. An early study by Khadem and colleagues demonstrated that DCE-MR imaging was able to distinguish spinal metastases from healthy bone marrow, in a retrospective analysis of 26 patients with spinal metastases, via comparison of overall TIC morphologies alone.[10] Spinal metastases demonstrated contrast enhancement above baseline, whereas healthy subjects showed minimal to no contrast enhancement (Type A: "flat" TIC[11]) (Fig. 2). Despite having similar appearance on conventional MR imaging, DCE-MR imaging can differentiate new spinal metastases from previously treated metastases.[10] DCE-MR imaging Vp heat maps and TIC can easily discriminate new metastases from treated metastases and from normal bone marrow (see Fig. 2).

Discriminating Hypervascular and Hypovascular Metastases

DCE-MR imaging can distinguish between hypervascular spinal metastases such as from renal cell carcinoma and hypovascular metastases such as from prostate carcinoma, whereas conventional MR imaging is simply unable to do so. Khadem and colleagues were able to demonstrate successful discrimination between hypervascular and hypovascular metastases using DCE-MR imaging semiquantitative methods.[10] Hypervascular metastases had higher average peak enhancement signal percentage change ($P < .01$) and higher average wash-in enhancement slope ($P < .01$) compared with hypovascular metastases.

Subsequently, Saha and colleagues demonstrated that hypervascular and hypovascular spinal metastases could also be distinguished quantitatively via DCE-MR imaging. In comparison to hypovascular spinal metastases, hypervascular metastases demonstrated higher Vp ($P < .001$) and Ktrans ($P < .01$) in keeping with expected increased neo-angiogenesis for hypervascular metastases. Hypervascular lesions had Vp values 1.8 times higher than hypovascular lesions, making Vp the best discriminator between the two groups.[15] The second-best discriminator was peak enhancement signal percentage change, which was 1.6 times higher for hypervascular spinal metastases.[15]

Furthermore, Mazura and colleagues demonstrated that DCE-MR imaging can serve as a noninvasive surrogate to catheter-directed digital subtraction imaging spinal angiography, for evaluation of tumor vascularity.[16] Thus, DCE-MR imaging can be used to determine hypervascularity noninvasively and direct preoperative tumor embolization to reduce intraoperative blood loss.[13]

Assessing Treatment Response Post-Radiation Therapy

In addition to diagnosing vertebral body metastases, DCE-MR imaging can also play a valuable role in monitoring posttreatment response, in patients who undergo radiotherapy. Although viable tumor demonstrates hyperperfusion due to neo-angiogenesis, radiation therapy induces alterations in tumor microvasculature that decrease blood flow secondary to induction of thrombosis, fibrosis, and apoptosis.[17] Lis and colleagues demonstrated that DCE-MR imaging can detect decreased perfusion 1 hour after high-dose image-guided radiation therapy.[8] Vp was reported to drop on average 65% ($P < .05$) 1 hour posttreatment when compared with pretreatment, and remained decreased on follow-up imaging, suggesting successful treatment[8] (see Fig. 2). Early reduction in Vp status post-radiation therapy has been established as the leading predictor of successful treatment response. In contradistinction,

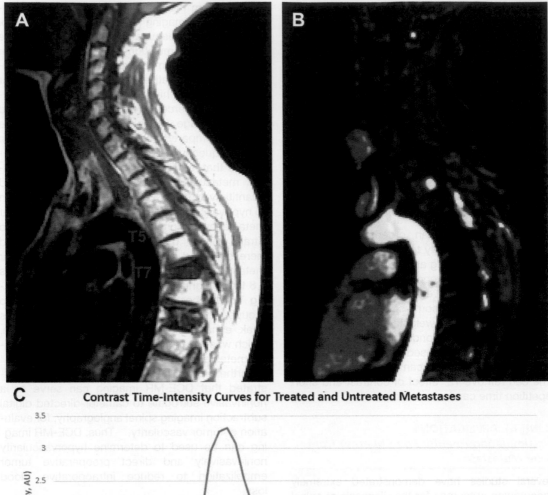

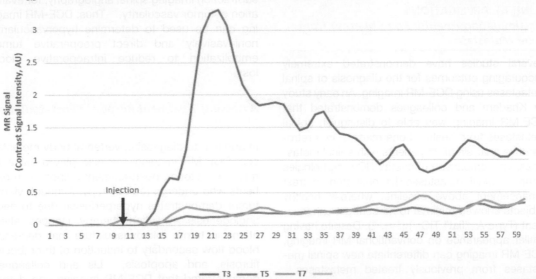

Fig. 2. Illustration of normal marrow, treated tumor and viable tumor. Sagittal T1 pre-contrast (*A*) image demonstrates a small metastasis in the posterior aspect of the T3 vertebral body, normal marrow signal of T5, and diffuse metastatic involvement of T7. Based on the routine MR sequences, including sagittal T1 (shown), inversion recovery (IR), T2 and post-contrast T1 (not shown), it is impossible to distinguish between active and successfully treated metastases. Perfusion imaging (*B*) demonstrates elevated plasma volume that correlates with the T3 metastatic deposit, suggestive of viable disease. No hyperperfusion is identified at T5 consistent with normal marrow, and no hyperperfusion at T7 consistent with treated tumor. Time intensity curves (*C*) demonstrate rapid wash-in and wash-out of contrast at T3 (Type D curve in blue) consistent with viable tumor, whereas normal marrow at T5 and treated tumor at T7 demonstrate relatively flat (Type A curves in *orange* and *yellow*, respectively) TIC.

a much longer time is required to establish a successful treatment response via conventional imaging, which can only establish a lack of structural changes such as stable or decreased tumor volume.[18] In addition to quantitative metrics, qualitative TIC analysis has also been shown to be a good classifier of post-radiotherapy treatment response. Successfully treated spinal metastases demonstrate Type E curve (rapid wash-in followed by second slow rise in contrast enhancement), whereas unsuccessfully treated disease demonstrates Type D curve (rapid wash-in followed by wash-out).[18] In addition, DCE-MR imaging has been shown to be able to successfully identify local spinal metastatic recurrence 6 months before conventional MR imaging, by demonstrating elevated Vp and Ktrans.[19]

Identifying Benign and Pathologic Vertebral Compression Fractures

Benign vertebral compression fractures are prevalent and often painful in the older population and usually due to osteoporosis.[20] Patients with an underlying malignancy can develop pathologic compressions fractures due to an underlying metastasis, which are often difficult to differentiate from benign fractures (osteoporotic vs pathologic). In addition, cancer patients are at increased risk for benign compression fractures due to common treatment plans such as radiation therapy, steroid utilization, hormone therapy, and chemotherapy which can alter osseous density and contribute to compression fractures.[21] Clearly, the ability to differentiate between benign and malignant compression fractures is paramount in a patient with cancer, as this can mean the difference between "no evidence of disease" in the case of a benign fracture and stage 4 disease in the case of a pathologic fracture. Unfortunately, malignant and benign fractures have comparable appearances on conventional MR imaging, which further complicates diagnosis.[22] DCE-MR imaging can differentiate between osteoporotic and pathologic vertebral body fractures via perfusion metrics (**Fig. 3**). Arevalo-Perez and colleagues. demonstrated that pathologic fractures possessed higher Vp, Ktrans, peak enhancement, and wash-in-slope when compared with nonmalignant fractures ($P < .01$).[21] DCE-MR imaging also demonstrated improved sensitivity in discriminating between acute and chronic vertebral body fractures.[23]

Recognizing Chordomas

Chordomas are a rare type of osseous spinal malignancy that is locally invasive, aggressive and

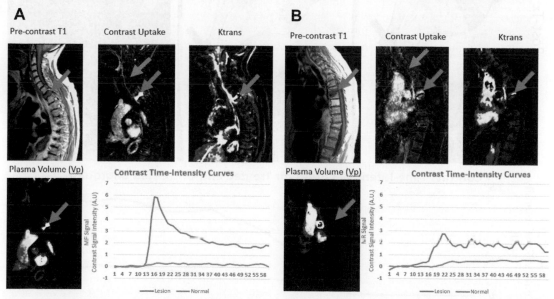

Fig. 3. Pathologic versus nonneoplastic compression fractures. (*A*) Sagittal T1 (*top left*) demonstrates hypointense marrow replacing T1 lesion (*blue arrow*) with vertebral height loss consistent with compression fracture and normal marrow (*oranage arrow*). In the setting of associated elevated plasma volume on perfusion imaging (*bottom left*) with Vp of 38, the finding is most consistent with viable metastasis with associated pathologic compression fracture. TIC (*bottom left* in *A*) also suggests metastasis with typical Type D curve in blue. (*B*) Sagittal T1 (*top right*) demonstrates hypointense T6 lesion (*blue arrow*) with mild vertebral height loss consistent with compression fracture and normal marrow (*oranage arrow*). There is no significant elevated plasma volume (Vp of 0.15) on perfusion imaging (*bottom right B*). Constellation of findings are consistent with nonneoplastic compression fracture.

has a poor prognosis.[24] They are also known to be prone to recurrence.[25] In addition, chordomas are difficult to assess for treatment response on conventional imaging, as they do not demonstrate significant change in anatomic appearance after positive treatment response to therapy. Adding to the difficulty is relative clinical indolence before

rapid progression and subsequent treatment resistance.[24] DCE-MR imaging has shown to successfully delineate effective treatment response from treatment failure, particularly via lower quantitative perfusion metrics such as Vp and Ktrans[26] (Fig. 4). In addition, chordomas have been shown to have a distinct Type E TIC characterized by

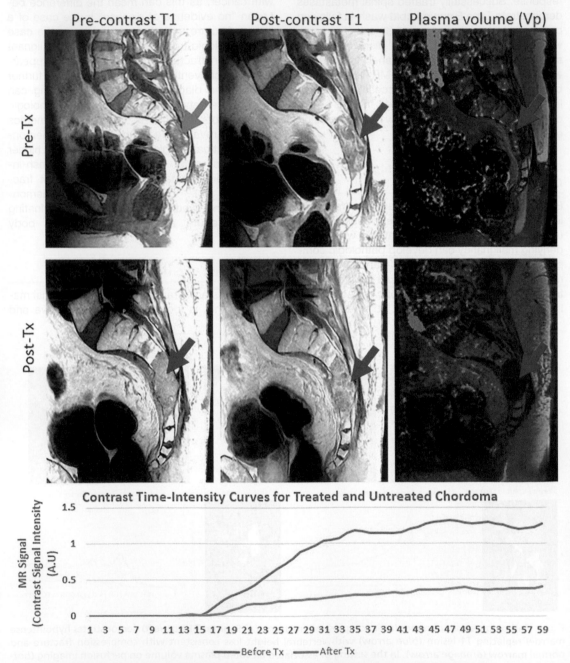

Fig. 4. Pretreatment and posttreatment assessment of chordoma. Pretreatment sagittal images (top row) demonstrate enhancing marrow replacing mass centered at S3–S4 (red and blue arrows) with associated hyperperfusion (Vp of 2.6). Posttreatment sagittal images illustrate similar heterogenous enhancing mass centered at S3–S4; however, there is a significant decrease in perfusion (dark on bottom right image) with Vp of 0.14, consistent with treatment response. TIC curves also demonstrate reduced TIC for treated disease.

rapid wash-in with subsequent second slow rise in contrast enhancement; thus, this may allow differentiation from other spinal lesions.[26]

Diagnosing Atypical Intraosseous Venous Malformations

Owing to their low-fat content and increased vascularity, atypical intraosseous venous malformations (also known as "hemangiomas") are common benign tumors that can at times resemble spinal metastasis or other neoplastic lesions on conventional MR imaging.[27] Morales and colleagues demonstrated that spinal metastases can be differentiated from atypical hemangiomas via DCE-MR imaging quantitative metrics, as spinal metastases show higher Ktrans ($P < .01$) and Vp ($P < .01$) values[28] (**Fig. 5**). Qualitative perfusion analysis also helps to discriminate between hemangiomas and spinal metastases, as the latter demonstrate increased signal intensities and Type D TIC (rapid wash-in followed by wash-out of contrast).[28]

APPLICATIONS TO EVERYDAY CLINICAL PRACTICE

DCE-MR imaging is an integral part of our practice with approximately 35% to 40% of our total MR

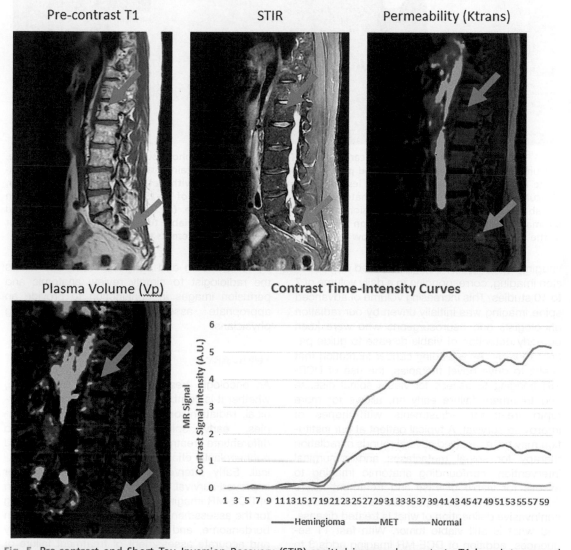

Pre-contrast T1 · STIR · Permeability (Ktrans)

Plasma Volume (Vp) · Contrast Time-Intensity Curves

— Hemingioma — MET — Normal

Fig. 5. Pre-contrast and Short Tau Inversion Recovery (STIR) sagittal images demonstrate T1 hypointense and mildly T2 hyperintense lesions in the L1 (*blue arrow*) and S2 (*orange arrow*) vertebral bodies. Perfusion imaging, however, shows elevated plasma volume in the S2 lesion of 13.5 which is suggestive of metastasis and reduced plasma volume in the L1 lesion of 0.2 which is suggestive of nonneoplastic etiology. Therefore, in conjunction with the anatomic appearance, the L1 lesion is most consistent with an atypical hemangioma. In addition, the S2 metastatic deposit demonstrates expected rapid wash-in on TIC (*bottom right*).

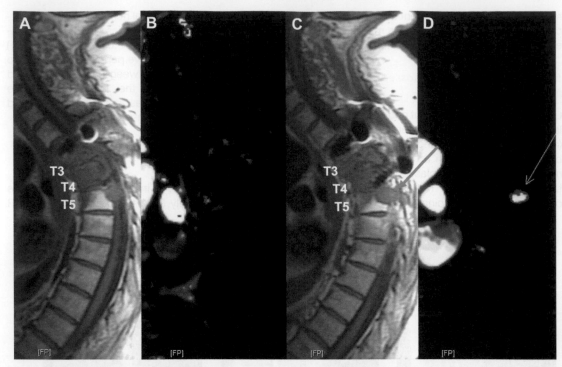

Fig. 6. Patient with metastatic thyroid carcinoma to T2–T5, status post-kyphoplasty for T3 pathologic fracture, instrumented stabilization of T2–T4, and post-radiation therapy. (A, C) Obtained several months apart, demonstrate T1 hypointense marrow replacing lesions involving T2–T5 consistent with metastatic disease. It is, however, difficult to delineate, simply based on anatomic imaging, which component of T2–T5 is treated disease and which is viable tumor. (B) No elevated perfusion consistent with treated disease. (D) On follow-up, shows elevated plasma volume in the posterior T5 lesion (green arrow), consistent with viable tumor, whereas the remainder of the correlative T1 hypointense marrow replacing lesion seen on 6C represents treated disease.

imaging spine volume being performed with perfusion imaging, corresponding to a daily volume of 7 to 10 studies. This increasing volume of advanced spine imaging was initially driven by our radiation oncologists and neurosurgeons who were keen on early detection of viable disease to guide patient therapy. As a leading cancer institution that seeks to drive novel therapies, the use of DCE-MR imaging to assess for viable spinal disease and treatment failure early on, allows for more rapid treatment adjustments with hopes of improving survival. A typical patient at our institution may have received several rounds of radiation therapy for spinal metastases and/or surgical intervention, confounding anatomic imaging to assess for viable disease and treatment failure (Fig. 6). DCE-MR imaging allows for accurate noninvasive delineation of what is treated disease, and what is still viable tumor. With fast T1 sequences, addition of DCE-MR imaging adds 3 to 4 minutes to a routine scan time. There are several software packages readily available to analyze perfusion data. At our institution, both Ktrans and Vp as well as overlayed perfusion on anatomic T1-weighted images are processed by a

dedicated team and sent to PACS. This allows the radiologist to simply review anatomic and perfusion images in conjunction to provide an appropriate assessment for the referring physicians.

SUMMARY

As oncologic treatments continue to advance, whether it is combination therapies (medical, surgical, radiation) or individualized targeted therapies, early spinal lesion assessment to differentiate treatment failure, viable tumor, and nonneoplastic etiology becomes increasingly critical. Early intervention in turn can allow for improved survival. In our experience, the addition of DCE-MR imaging to conventional MR imaging for the assessment of spinal lesions has not been burdensome, and in fact has allowed for early and accurate assessment of treatment failure or viable tumor, information that is exceedingly helpful for our referring radiation oncologists and neurosurgeons. DCE-MR imaging has become a mainstay in our clinical spinal neuro-oncological practice.

CLINICS CARE POINTS

- Spinal metastases demonstrate elevated plasma volume (Vp) and permeability constant (Ktrans) on DCE-MR imaging, indicative of viable tumor.
- Reduced quantitative perfusion parameters are suggestive of treatment response and nonviable disease.
- Hypervascular metastases demonstrate increased elevated perfusion parameters when compared with hypovascular metastases.
- Atypical intraosseous venous malformation (benign lesion) does not demonstrate elevated perfusion when compared with spinal metastases
- Vertebral body compression deformities with elevated Vp and Ktrans are likely pathologic.

DISCLOSURE

A.I. Holodny is the owner and President of fMRI Consultants, LLC, the work of which is not related to this article. The other authors have nothing to disclose.

REFERENCES

1. Berg KD, Thomsen FB, Mikkelsen MK, et al. Improved survival for patients with de novo metastatic prostate cancer in the last 20 years. Eur J Cancer 2017;72:20–7.

2. Perrin RG. Metastatic tumors of the axial spine. Curr Opin Oncol 1992;4(3):525–32.

3. Montazel JL, Divine M, Lepage E, et al. Normal Spinal Bone Marrow in Adults: Dynamic Gadolinium-enhanced MR Imaging. Radiology 2003;229(3):703–9.

4. Maccauro G, Spinelli MS, Mauro S, et al. Physiopathology of Spine Metastasis. International Journal of Surgical Oncology 2011;2011:107969.

5. Arevalo-Perez J, Peck KK, Young RJ, et al. Dynamic Contrast-Enhanced Perfusion MRI and Diffusion-Weighted Imaging in Grading of Gliomas. J Neuroimaging 2015;25(5):792–8.

6. Thomas AA, Arevalo-Perez J, Kaley T, et al. Dynamic contrast enhanced T1 MRI perfusion differentiates pseudoprogression from recurrent glioblastoma. J Neuro Oncol 2015;125(1):183–90.

7. Saha A, Peck KK, Lis E, et al. Magnetic Resonance Perfusion Characteristics of Hypervascular Renal and Hypovascular Prostate Spinal Metastases. Spine 2014;39(24):E1433–40.

8. Lis E, Saha A, Peck KK, et al. Dynamic contrast-enhanced magnetic resonance imaging of osseous spine metastasis before and 1 hour after high-dose image-guided radiation therapy. Neurosurg Focus 2017;42(1):E9.

9. Tofts PS, Brix G, Buckley DL, et al. Estimating kinetic parameters from dynamic contrast-enhanced T(1)-weighted MRI of a diffusable tracer: standardized quantities and symbols. J Magn Reson Imaging 1999;10(3):223–32.

10. Khadem NR, Karimi S, Peck KK, et al. Characterizing hypervascular and hypovascular metastases and normal bone marrow of the spine using dynamic contrast-enhanced MR imaging. AJNR Am J Neuroradiol 2012;33(11):2178–85.

11. Chen WT, Shih TTF, Chen RC, et al. Blood perfusion of vertebral lesions evaluated with gadolinium-enhanced dynamic MRI: in comparison with compression fracture and metastasis. J Magn Reson Imaging 2002;15(3):308–14.

12. Galbraith SM, Lodge MA, Taylor NJ, et al. Reproducibility of dynamic contrast-enhanced MRI in human muscle and tumours: comparison of quantitative and semi-quantitative analysis. NMR Biomed 2002;15(2):132–42.

13. Walker-Samuel S, Leach MO, Collins DJ. Evaluation of response to treatment using DCE-MRI: the relationship between initial area under the gadolinium curve (IAUGC) and quantitative pharmacokinetic analysis. Phys Med Biol 2006;51(14):3593–602.

14. Saranathan M, Rettmann DW, Hargreaves BA, et al. DIfferential Subsampling with Cartesian Ordering (DISCO): a high spatio-temporal resolution Dixon imaging sequence for multiphasic contrast enhanced abdominal imaging. J Magn Reson Imaging 2012;35(6):1484–92.

15. Saha A, Peck KK, Lis E, et al. Magnetic resonance perfusion characteristics of hypervascular renal and hypovascular prostate spinal metastases: clinical utilities and implications: Clinical utilities and implications. Spine 2014;39(24):E1433–40.

16. Mazura JC, Karimi S, Pauliah M, et al. Dynamic contrast–enhanced magnetic resonance perfusion compared with digital subtraction angiography for the evaluation of extradural spinal metastases: A pilot study. Spine 2014;39(16):E950–4.

17. Barker HE, Paget JTE, Khan AA, et al. Erratum: The tumour microenvironment after radiotherapy: mechanisms of resistance and recurrence. Nat Rev Cancer 2015;15(8):509.

18. Chu S, Karimi S, Peck KK, et al. Measurement of blood perfusion in spinal metastases with dynamic contrast-enhanced magnetic resonance imaging: Evaluation of tumor response to radiation therapy. Spine 2013;38(22):E1418–24.

19. Kumar KA, Peck KK, Karimi S, et al. A pilot study evaluating the use of dynamic contrast-enhanced

perfusion MRI to predict local recurrence after radio-surgery on spinal metastases. Technol Cancer Res Treat 2017;16(6):857–65.

20. Jung HS, Jee WH, McCauley TR, et al. Discrimination of metastatic from acute osteoporotic compression spinal fractures with MR imaging. Radiographics 2003;23(1):179–87.

21. Croarkin E. Osteopenia in the patient with cancer. Phys Ther 1999;79(2):196–201.

22. Verstraete KL, Van der Woude HJ, Hogendoorn PC, et al. Dynamic contrast-enhanced MR imaging of musculoskeletal tumors: basic principles and clinical applications. J Magn Reson Imaging 1996; 6(2):311–21.

23. Arevalo-Perez J, Peck KK, Lyo JK, et al. Differentiating benign from malignant vertebral fractures using T1-weighted dynamic contrast-enhanced MRI: Differentiating Benign, Malignant Fractures. J Magn Reson Imaging 2015;42(4):1039–47.

24. Walcott BP, Nahed BV, Mohyeldin A, et al. Chordoma: current concepts, management, and future directions. Lancet Oncol 2012;13(2):e69–76.

25. Bergh P, Kindblom LG, Gunterberg B, et al. Prognostic factors in chordoma of the sacrum and mobile spine: A study of 39 patients. Cancer 2000;88(9): 2122–34.

26. Santos P, Peck KK, Arevalo-Perez J, et al. T1-weighted dynamic contrast-enhanced MR perfusion imaging characterizes tumor response to radiation therapy in chordoma. Am J Neuroradiol 2017; 38(11):2210–6.

27. Gaudino S, Martucci M, Colantonio R, et al. A systematic approach to vertebral hemangioma. Skeletal Radiol 2015;44(1):25–36.

28. Morales KA, Arevalo-Perez J, Peck KK, et al. Differentiating atypical hemangiomas and metastatic vertebral lesions: The role of T1-weighted dynamic contrast-enhanced MRI. Am J Neuroradiol 2018; 39(5):968–73.

Management Algorithm for Osseous Metastatic Disease: What the Treatment Teams Want to Know

Wende N. Gibbs, MD, MA[a,*], Mahmud Mossa Basha, MD[b],
J. Levi Chazen, MD[c]

KEYWORDS

- Spine • Oncology • Metastatic disease • SBRT • Spine surgery • Advanced imaging
- Spinal instability neoplastic score • SINS

KEY POINTS

- Radiologists play a primary role in identifying, characterizing, and classifying spinal metastases and can play a lifesaving role in the care of these patients by triaging those with instability to urgent spine surgery consultation.
- Evidence-based management algorithms, such as NOMS, serve as frameworks to guide discussion, suggesting treatment options based on the most current literature and options. Approximately 50% of the information in NOMS is obtained from the patient's images and radiology report.
- The radiologist should report the spinal instability neoplastic score and epidural spinal cord compression grade to ensure clear communication and timely, appropriate patient care.
- Advances in imaging, such as synthetic CT, dynamic contrast-enhanced perfusion MR imaging, and dynamic cord imaging, will provide more precise characterization of pathology and improved patient safety.

INTRODUCTION

The spine is the most common site of skeletal metastases, affecting approximately 40% of patients with cancer.[1] Up to 20% of these will become symptomatic due to spinal cord compression, suffering from severe pain, loss of function, paralysis, or death.[2,3] Cord compression may result from pathologic fracture with retropulsion of bone into the canal or from epidural extension of disease. Radiologists play a primary role in identifying, characterizing, and classifying spinal metastases and can play a lifesaving role in the care of

these patients by triaging those with instability to urgent spine surgery consultation. For this reason, an understanding of current treatment algorithms and principles of spinal stability in patients with cancer is vital for all who interpret spine studies. In addition, advances in imaging allow radiologists to provide more accurate diagnoses and characterize pathology, thereby improving patient safety. This article discusses current classification schemes in spine oncology and advanced imaging approaches that provide pathophysiological information instrumental to treatment planning and prognosis

[a] Barrow Neurological Institute, Department of Neuroradiology, St. Joseph's Hospital and Medical Center, 350 West Thomas Road, Phoenix, AZ 85013, USA; [b] University of Washington School of Medicine, 1959 Northeast Pacific Street, Seattle, WA 98195, USA; [c] Hospital for Special Surgery, 535 East 70th Street, New York, NY 10021, USA
* Corresponding author. 18522 North 96th Way, Scottsdale, AZ 85255.
E-mail address: Wende.Gibbs@BarrowNeuro.Org

Neuroimag Clin N Am 33 (2023) 487–497
https://doi.org/10.1016/j.nic.2023.04.003
1052-5149/23/© 2023 Elsevier Inc. All rights reserved.

SPINE ONCOLOGY: MULTIDISCIPLINARY MANAGEMENT

The goals of treatment for spinal metastases include pain palliation, local durable pain control, maintenance or recovery of neurologic function and ambulation, mechanical stability, and improved quality of life. The principal methods of treatment include surgery and radiation therapy. Radiotherapy is often the initial treatment, because it is the most effective and least invasive modality for local tumor control.[4] Surgery is indicated for spinal instability and deformity, progressive neurological deficits, cord or nerve root compression by epidural disease or retropulsed bone, or treatment of metastases for which radiotherapy cannot safely be delivered. Surgical treatment may involve decompression alone or may include stabilization. Immunotherapy, chemotherapy, radionuclide, and hormone therapy may also play a role in treatment. Percutaneous cement augmentation and tumor ablation are increasingly used interventions in patients with painful metastases without cord compression.

Treatment of patients with cancer and spinal osseous metastatic disease is a multidisciplinary effort. Evidence-based management algorithms serve as frameworks to guide discussion, suggesting treatment options based on the most current literature and options. The most well-known is the NOMS framework devised at Memorial Sloan Kettering,[4] which takes into account patient factors including neurological status, oncologic status, mechanical spinal stability, and overall systemic status. These aspects of the patient's condition are used to guide systemic and radiation therapy, surgery, and nonsurgical spinal stabilization based on patient's specific characteristics and needs.

The neurological status includes the degree of spinal cord compression, myelopathy, and radiculopathy caused by osseous or soft tissue impingement on the spinal cord and nerve roots. The oncologic status is based on the tumor histology, chemosensitivity, hormonal sensitivity, and radiosensitivity to external beam radiation. Mechanical instability in the setting of metastatic disease is defined as "… the loss of spinal integrity as a result of a neoplastic process that is associated with movement related pain, symptomatic or progressive deformity, and/or neural compromise under physiologic loads."[5] An unstable spine must be treated with surgery regardless of the other aspects of the patient's status. Systemic status includes patient comorbidities, current health status, and the ability to tolerate surgery.

THE RADIOLOGIST'S ROLE IN ASSESSMENT

At least 50% of the information going into this decision-making process is obtained from the patient's images and radiology report.[4] Radiologists should be familiar with the management frameworks and language used by the treatment team to provide efficient, effective communication. The two most important scales for the radiologist to include in the radiology report are the spinal instability neoplastic score (SINS),[5] which characterizes mechanical stability, and the epidural spinal cord compression scale (ESCC),[6] which addresses the neurologic status of the patient.

THE SPINAL INSTABILITY NEOPLASTIC SCORE

Mechanical instability is an indication for surgical stabilization or percutaneous cement augmentation, regardless of neurologic or oncologic assessments; radiation therapy cannot stabilize an unstable spine. This determination is based on imaging and clinical examination. Radiologists play a primary role in triaging patients with an unstable spine to surgical consultation; timely triage is vital to prevent the catastrophic consequences of spinal failure in the setting of metastatic disease.

The SINS classification system allows for assessment of current and potential instability. SINS was devised and validated by the Spine Oncology Study Group in 2010 and was quickly adopted by multiple specialties caring for spine oncology patients. SINS characterizes spinal stability by answering six multiple choice questions and assigning point values to the answer options (Fig. 1). There are five radiographic features evaluated on MR imaging or computed tomography (CT) and one clinical component. The total score ranges from 0 to 18 with higher scores suggesting an unstable or potentially unstable spine. The five radiologic features include location of the metastasis in the spine, spinal alignment, lesion quality (lytic, sclerotic, or mixed), the degree of vertebral body involvement and collapse, and involvement of the posterior elements. The clinical component is mechanical back pain. This is a unique characteristic of oncologic instability compared with instability from other etiologies such as trauma or degenerative change; therefore, the assessment of mechanical back pain is necessary to provide a complete SINS score. The radiologist may not have this information but can still report the remaining parameters with this caveat for final grading by the treatment team. A high SINS score, 13 to 18, indicates the need for urgent surgical consultation and possible intervention. The indeterminate category, score of 7 to 12 should prompt

Questions	Answers (Point assignment)				
	4	3	2	1	0
Location		Junctional	Mobile	Semi-rigid	Rigid
Quality			Lytic	Mixed	Blastic
Alignment	Subluxation		Deformity		Preserved
Collapse		>50%	<50%	<50% but >50% body involved	None
Posterior Elements		Bilateral		Unilateral	None
Pain (Mechanical)		Yes		Occasional, not mechanical	No
Score	13–18 = Unstable		7–12 = Indeterminate	0–6 = Stable	
Recommendation	Urgent surgical consult		Surgical consult		

Fig. 1. Components of the spinal instability neoplastic score (SINS).

surgical consultation as quickly as possible. A score of 1 to 6 suggests that currently the spine is stable, and treatment planning for the cancer can be carried out with less concern for performing immediate spinal stabilization.

When evaluating spinal metastases, only the most unstable level matters for determining the urgency of spine surgery consultation. Evaluating all involved levels that may need to be addressed in the short term is beneficial for the treatment team. For each level, the six multiple choice questions should be answered with the choices provided in the system. Whether or not the radiologist provides a final score, describing these features is beneficial for quickly determining spinal stability. In addition, using language familiar to the treatment team that can also be used for research across institutions may further refine the algorithms and optimize patient care (Fig. 2).

At Which Level Is the Metastasis?

The consequences of spinal column failure depend on the level. Junctional levels, such as the craniocervical and cervicothoracic junctions, have the greatest mechanical stresses, and a lower burden of disease is necessary for failure. These levels are assigned the highest number of points for this category. The thoracic levels have extra stabilization from the ribs, so a larger volume of disease at any given level is required before column failure occurs. Fracture/spinal failure of the sacral levels will produce less profound effects than other levels and is assigned a lower number of points.

What Is the Alignment?

Normal alignment is not assigned any points. Loss of alignment, whether frank subluxation, an indicator of current instability, or new kyphosis or scoliosis, suggesting impending instability are assigned four and two points, respectively.

Are the Posterior Elements Involved?

In the lumbar spine, the pedicles are important stabilizers, whereas in the thoracic spine, the costovertebral joints are vital, given the extra stabilization provided by the ribs and sternum. Involvement of these structures receives three points if bilateral and one point if unilateral.

What Is the Lesion Quality?

Lytic metastases are more likely to collapse than blastic lesions, though both have compromised, abnormal bone. Lytic metastases receive two points, blastic lesions no points, and mixed lesions, which are indeterminate, receive one point.

What Is the Volume of Body Involved or the Degree of Collapse?

Pathologic fracture creates instability. This component of the system classifies degree of collapse into four categories: greater than 50%, which receives three points, less than 50%, which gets two points, no collapse but greater than 50% body involvement, which receives one point, and no collapse, which is assigned no points.

Does the Patient Have Mechanical Back Pain?

Mechanical pain is the single clinical component of the system. Pain with movement or axial loading of the spine, which is relieved by recumbence, is typical of mechanical pain. This differs from the pain associated with neoplastic involvement of the bone, which produces inflammatory factors and periosteal stretch. This biologic pain responds to steroids and radiation, whereas mechanical pain does not.[7] The two types of pain may coexist, but for the purpose of assessing potential instability, the mechanical pain receives the highest number of points. Nonmechanical or occasional pain is given a lower score.

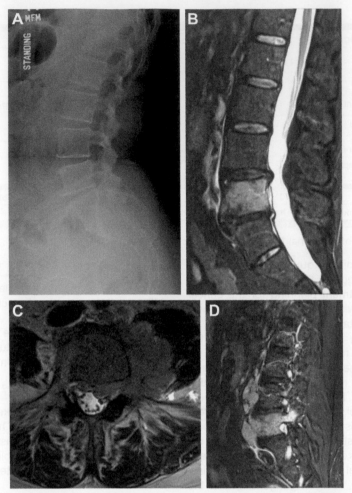

Fig. 2. Application of the SINS score. A 45-year-old woman consulted the pain clinic for a severe and increasing left leg radiculopathy. She had no significant medical history. The lateral radiograph (*A*) appeared normal. Sagittal STIR (*B*) and axial T2-weighted (*C*) images show marrow signal abnormality of the L5 vertebral body, with large associated soft tissue mass extending into the left neural foramen and into the anterior epidural space, accounting for the patient's symptoms. An off-midline sagittal T1-weighted fat-saturated post-contrast image (*D*) shows involvement of one pedicle. Her SINS score is nine (Location: L5, junctional, 3pts; Lesion quality: mixed [not sclerotic or lytic on CT], 1pt; Alignment: normal, 0pts; Volume/Collapse: no collapse, greater than 50% involved, 1pt; Posterior element involvement: unilateral, 1pt; Pain: severe mechanical, 3pts). A score of nine is indeterminate and the patient was seen by spine surgery for stability evaluation. pt, point; pts, points.

The SINS score is a useful source of information for devising an individualized plan for the patient using NOMS principles. However, it is also important in settings such as the emergency room or urgent care center, where patients may present with unknown metastatic disease, known cancer with new metastases, or treated disease with new recurrence. In these situations, it can be vital to make the ordering physician aware of spinal instability and the need for prompt surgical consultation.

THE EPIDURAL SPINAL CORD COMPRESSION SCALE

Prompt recognition of cord compression due to epidural extension of disease is vital for preservation

of neurological function. Standardized reporting of the degree of cord compression is necessary for effective communication with the treatment team and the key decision branch point that leads directly to radiation treatment or to a combination of minimally invasive surgery and radiation. The six-point ESCC is used in conjunction with clinical assessment of myelopathy and/or radiculopathy for these treatment decisions.[4,6] Grading is performed on axial T2-weighted images at the site of greatest compression. Grade 0 is a metastasis confined to the bone. Grade 1 is given to disease extending into the epidural space without cord compression. Grade 2 is epidural disease compressing the cord with some volume of preserved cerebrospinal fluid

(CSF). Grade 3 is epidural disease compressing the cord, obliterating the CSF (Fig. 3). If the spine is mechanically stable, radiation is considered for initial treatment in patients with low-grade cord compression (ESCC grades 0 and 1). High-grade compression (Grades 2 and 3) requires initial minimally invasive surgical decompression of tumor in the epidural space before going to radiation treatment. The exception to this approach includes highly radiosensitive tumor types (ie, lymphoma, myeloma, seminoma), for which a patient will receive primary radiation treatment, regardless of cord compression or neurologic deficit, or patients who cannot tolerate surgery.[4]

Rational for utilization of the ESCC in spine oncology is based on current treatment methods. Traditionally, osseous spinal metastases were treated with extensive surgeries with en bloc resections that resulted in substantial morbidity and provided poor long-term control. Alternatively, conventional external beam radiotherapy (cEBRT) was used for pain and tumor control in the relatively small set of histologies responsive to this treatment. The development and increasing use of stereotactic body radiotherapy (SBRT) has changed the treatment paradigm. cEBRT is typically delivered using two opposed beams with near full-dose radiation across the entire width of the patient. For this reason, doses must be kept low within tolerance of the most sensitive structures, such as the spinal cord. In contrast, SBRT/ stereotactic radiosurgery (SRS) is a highly conformal therapy using multiple beams or arcs focused on the tumor target with a steep dose fall-off, allowing for a high, ablative dose in one

to five fractions. Tumors that were moderately sensitive or not sensitive to cEBRT are nearly all sensitive to SBRT with very high rates of tumor control. This has made radiotherapy the first-line treatment for osseous spinal metastases in most cases. In situations where there is ESCC Grade 0 or 1, SBRT can be used to target the tumor in bone with sufficient dose to the epidural component. In cases of high ESCC Grades 2 and 3, separation surgery, a smaller procedure to remove the epidural component of tumor before the bulk is treated with radiation, is performed first (Fig. 4).

THE FUTURE OF NOMS AND SINS: RADIOLOGY INNOVATION

Spine oncology treatments continue to advance. Radiology will always play a vital role in the multidisciplinary care of these patients. Radiology images and reports are vital components in radiomic modeling and predictive data analysis. Although this is still in the preclinical stage, radiologists can work to standardize image protocols and reports to enable more accurate and reproducible algorithms.[8] Additional areas of innovation in radiology that will benefit patients with cancer include characterization of patient frailty, improved prediction of recurrence and fracture, and novel techniques that will improve patient safety and lesion characterization.

SYSTEMIC STATUS (FRAILTY) BODY COMPOSITION

Systemic status is a clinical factor that has not traditionally been within the purview of radiology.

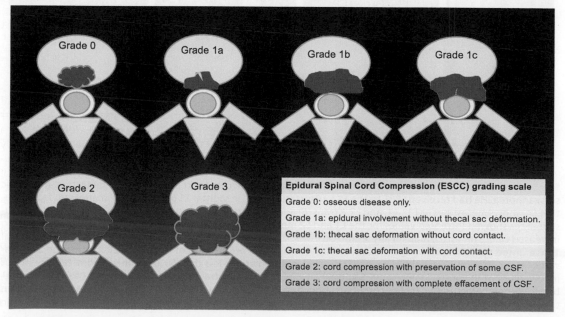

Fig. 3. Assessment using the epidural spinal cord compression scale (ESCC).

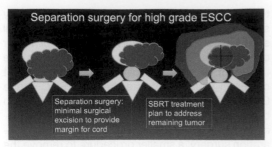

Fig. 4. Explanation of separation surgery in the setting of high-grade cord compression.

However, the importance of frailty and sarcopenia is increasingly recognized for predicting survival and postoperative complications, therefore, a vital component of treatment decision-making. CT-based body composition measures have been shown to improve preoperative risk assessment as surrogate markers for frailty. Sarcopenia, muscle density, visceral fat and subcutaneous fat volumes, and ratios have been correlated with outcomes in a number of specific cancer types and after spinal surgery for osseous metastatic disease.[9–11]

DYNAMIC CONTRAST-ENHANCED MR IMAGING

Advanced imaging techniques have been used to improve detection and classification of tumor as well as to predict recurrence and posttreatment complications such as vertebral compression fracture. Dynamic contrast-enhanced (DCE) MR imaging has shown promise in differentiating benign from malignant marrow processes and evaluating tumor response to radiation therapy.[12] DCE perfusion can also predict future recurrence post-SBRT, relative to local control, and 6 months earlier than conventional MR imaging.[13] (Fig. 5).

DCE data can be processed semiquantitatively using dynamic changes during passage of the

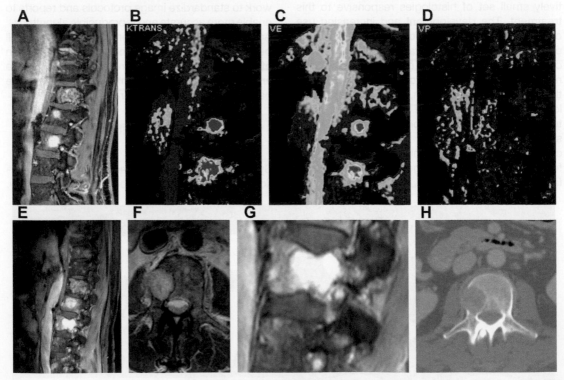

Fig. 5. Prediction of disease recurrence with MR imaging DCE perfusion in a patient with metastatic melanotic schwannoma. He had received SBRT to the T12 metastasis only. The sagittal T1 post-contrast image with fat saturation (A) shows metastases at T12, L1, and L2. Ktrans (B) and Ve (extravascular extracellular coefficient) (C) DCE perfusion maps showed increased values for the L1 and L2 metastatic lesions, but not for the T12 lesion. There were no increased values on Vp (D) map for any lesion. On 6-week follow-up, the T12 metastasis appears stable in the sagittal T1-weighted post-contrast image (E). There is however interval progression of the L1 and L2 lesions. The L2 metastatic lesion on axial T2-weighted image (F) showed involvement of less than 50% of the vertebral body, without involvement of the posterior elements. Sagittal T1-weighted post-contrast image (G) indicates less than 50% vertebral body height loss, but no scoliosis or subluxation. Axial post-contrast CT (H) shows that the lesion is lytic. Based on these factors, the spine instability neoplastic score (SINS) ranged from 6 to 9, depending on pain symptoms.

contrast bolus that are depicted as time–intensity curves. In this scenario, perfusion values such as peak-enhancement, wash-in, and wash-out can be obtained. Myeloma and metastatic lesions often have curves with rapid wash-in (with or without wash-out), whereas posttreatment changes demonstrate slow wash-in with a persistent or plateau course of enhancement.[14] The absolute quantification of DCE data can be performed using mathematical modeling that depicts changes in tissue contrast concentrations instead of signal intensity changes over time. Perfusion values such as permeability (Ktrans) and plasma volume (Vp)

have shown promising results in the evaluation of posttreatment changes[15] (Fig. 6).

SYNTHETIC CT

Synthetic CT is an exciting development which may someday help surgeons decrease the number of imaging studies, decrease patient radiation dose, and improve characterization of metastases. Recent innovations in cortical bone imaging have enabled MR imaging-generated images with CT-like contrast, commonly referred to as bone MR imaging or synthetic CT. Cortical bone has a very

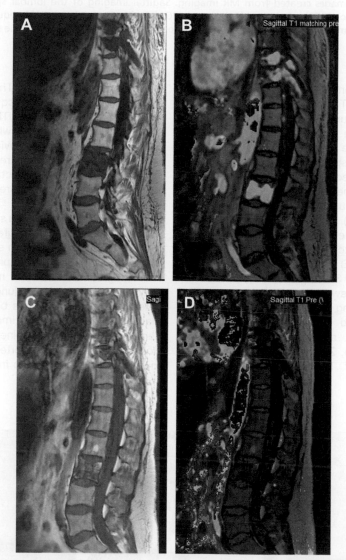

Fig. 6. Value of MR imaging perfusion evaluation of treatment efficacy. Sagittal T1-weighted image (*A*) shows multiple active, T1-hypointense metastatic bone lesions from breast cancer, in the thoracic and lumbar spine. On the DCE perfusion (*B*) image, these lesions demonstrate elevated plasma volume (*Vp*). Four months following radiation therapy, the metastases are still T1-hypointense (*C*), but the plasma volume has normalized (*D*), indicating successful treatment. (*Courtesy of* J Tisnado, MD, New York, NY).

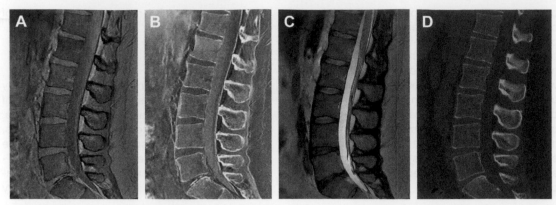

Fig. 7. Synthetic CT images created from MR imaging. Sagittal imaging of the lumbar spine using a spoiled gradient recalled echo (SPGR) sequence (*A*), inverted SPGR (*B*), 3D T2-weighted CUBE sequence (*C*), and corresponding sagittal CT image (*D*). Note the cortical detail from the "synthetic CT" in *B* and the similarity to standard CT imaging in *D*.

short T2 relaxation on the order of 0.1 to 1 ms, and standard spin-echo T1- and T2-weighted pulse sequences fail to capture cortical bone signal due to signal decay before radiofrequency ablation (RF) readout.[16] To image the very short T2 relaxation of cortical bone, specialized pulse sequences have been developed including ultrashort time to echo (UTE), zero time to echo (ZTE), and modified gradient echo and susceptibility-weighted imaging (SWI) (Figs. 7 and 8).

ZTE pulse sequences activate the readout gradient before excitation, thereby decreasing the time to echo (TE) as close to zero as possible. ZTE is an inherently 3D sequence and, due to the lack of gradient switching, can be used to perform MR imaging with decreased acoustical noise for improved patient comfort. Because k-space sampling starts with the gradients already ramped up, ZTE suffers from data loss in the center of k-space with associated decreased image contrast. This can be compensated for by oversampled acquisitions and mathematical reconstructions. UTE uses a short RF pulse for signal excitation, whereas the readout gradient is ramped up, achieving TEs on the order of 8 to 50 μs. UTE provides greater flexibility in image contrast by a larger spectrum of available flip angles but suffers from increased eddy current and chemical shift artifacts.[17]

In the spine, UTE has been studied for detection of pars interarticularis fractures in cadavers with near perfect agreement with standard CT.[18] UTE has also been described in spine trauma, showing robust agreement with CT measurements.[19] In addition, the craniocervical junction has been evaluated with UTE.[20] SWI has become a commonplace sequence for brain imaging but has also demonstrated value for spine oncology imaging. Böker and colleagues reported the ability of SWI to differentiate osteoblastic from osteolytic spine

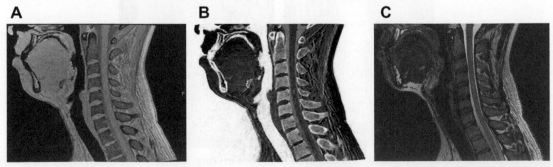

Fig. 8. Synthetic CT images of the cervical spine. Sagittal image created using a spoiled gradient recalled echo (SPGR) sequence (*A*), inverted SPGR (*B*), and corresponding T2-weighted sequence (*C*). Note the "CT-like" contrast of cortical bone in B. The airway and ligamentum flavum appear bright on the inverted sequence, not to be confused with ligamentous mineralization.

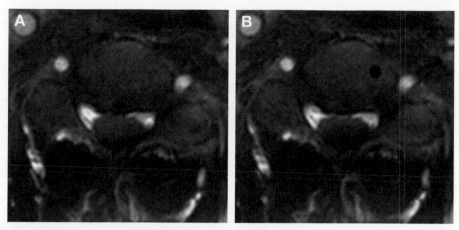

Fig. 9. Dynamic imaging of spinal cord motion in radiation therapy planning. Dynamic axial BFFE imaging shows contact between the anterior cervical spinal cord and the lesion in the ventral epidural space, on one frame (*A*), with a gap of 0.9 mm on a later frame (*B*).

metastases on MR imaging, an important distinction for interventional and radiotherapy planning.[21] Quantitative imaging of bone density has also been described with MR imaging techniques, potentially complementing or obviating the need for traditional nuclear medicine or quantitative CT-based bone density evaluation.[22]

IMAGING SPINAL CORD MOTION

Radiation treatment planning of the spinal column typically considers the spinal cord as a static structure; however, the spinal cord moves in an oscillatory pattern, corresponding to the cardiac cycle. The spinal cord moves in anterior–posterior, cranio-caudal, and right-to-left planes; however, the degree of motion differs based on the anatomic level.[23,24] One study indicated that the anterior–posterior cord motion was the most dramatic in the cervical and upper thoracic spine, with maximum displacement up to 0.64 mm, but attenuated in the thoracic spine below T4.[23] Spinal cord motion is most pronounced in the craniocaudal direction, followed by anterior–posterior, then left-to-right motion.[25] Spinal cord motion and its impact on treatment planning have recently received increased attention.[25,26] Treatment planning for SBRT using static spinal cord imaging can result in increased radiation dose to the cord of 0.6% to 13.8% (mean 4.3%) compared with dynamic imaging with exact cord positioning, and cord excursion beyond the static cord contours extended as much as 1.5 mm.[26]

Spinal cord motion can be accurately depicted with phase-contrast MR imaging[27,28] or cardiac-gated 3D dynamic balanced fast-field echo (BFFE) sequences[26] (**Fig. 9**).

SUMMARY

Radiologists who read spine imaging studies should be familiar with the NOMS framework to understand the vital role of the specialty in the care of patients with cancer. Utilization of the SINS and epidural spinal cord compression scale facilitates improved communication and patient care. As cancer care advances, so too does imaging science, allowing for more precise characterization of pathology and improved patient safety. The increasingly multidisciplinary management of these patients, and consideration of all factors which influence their care, outcomes, and quality of life, should prompt radiologists to learn more about innovations in the field that can contribute to this goal.[29]

CLINICS CARE POINTS

- Spinal instability in the setting of osseous metastatic disease requires prompt evaluation by a spine surgeon, as spinal column failure can produce more rapid deleterious effects than the patient's malignancy.

- CT characterization of sarcopenia, muscle density, visceral fat and subcutaneous fat volumes, and ratios have been correlated with outcomes in a number of specific cancer types and after spinal surgery for osseous metastatic disease.

- Quantitative imaging of bone density is possible with MR imaging techniques, potentially obviating the need for traditional nuclear medicine or quantitative CT based bone density evaluation with their inherent radiation dose to the patient.

DISCLOSURE

No disclosures for any author.

REFERENCES

1. Siegel RL, Miller KD, Fuchs HE, et al. Cancer statistics, 2022. CA Cancer J Clin 2022;72:7–33.
2. Barzilai O, Laufer I, Yamada Y, et al. Integrating Evidence-Based Medicine for Treatment of Spinal Metastases Into a Decision Framework: Neurologic, Oncologic, Mechanicals Stability, and Systemic Disease. J Clin Oncol 2017;35(21):2419–27.
3. Kaloostian PE, Yurter A, Zadnik PL, et al. Current paradigms for metastatic spinal disease: an evidence-based review. Ann Surg Oncol 2014; 21(1):248–62.
4. Laufer I, Rubin DG, Lis E, et al. The NOMS framework: approach to the treatment of spinal metastatic tumors. Oncol 2013;18(6):744–51.
5. Fisher CG, DiPaola CP, Ryken TC, et al. A novel classification system for spinal instability in neoplastic disease: an evidence-based approach and expert consensus from the Spine Oncology Study Group. Spine 2010;35:E1221–9.
6. Bilsky MH, Laufer I, Fourney DR, et al. Reliability analysis of the epidural spinal cord compression scale. J Neurosurg Spine 2010;13(3):324–8.
7. Posner JB. Back pain and epidural spinal cord compression. Med Clin North Am 1987;71:185–205.
8. Gui C, Chen X, Sheikh K, et al. Radiomic modeling to predict risk of vertebral compression fracture after stereotactic body radiation therapy for spinal metastases. J Neurosurg Spine 2021;1–9. https://doi.org/10.3171/2021.3.SPINE201534.
9. Lee MH, Pickhardt SG, Garrett JW, et al. Utility of fully automated body composition measures on pretreatment abdominal CT for predicting survival in patients with colorectal cancer. AJR Am J Roentgenol 2023;220(3):371–80.
10. Bates DDB, Pickhardt PJ. Ct-derived body composition assessment as a prognostic tool in oncologic patients: from opportunistic research to artificial intelligence-based clinical implementation. AJR Am J Roentgenol 2022;219(4):671–80.
11. Massaad E, Bridge CP, Kiapour A, et al. Evaluating frailty, mortality, and complications associated with metastatic spine tumor surgery using machine learning-derived body composition analysis. J Neurosurg Spine 2022;1–11. https://doi.org/10.3171/2022.1.SPINE211284.
12. Lang N, Su MY, Yu HJ, et al. Differentiation of myeloma and metastatic cancer in the spine using dynamic contrast-enhanced MRI. Magn Reson Imaging 2013;31(8):1285–91.
13. Kumar KA, Peck KK, Karimi S, et al. A pilot study evaluating the use of dynamic contrast-enhanced perfusion MRI to predict local recurrence after radiosurgery on spinal metastases. Technol Cancer Res Treat 2017;16(6):857–65.
14. Cao Y. The promise of dynamic contrast-enhanced imaging in radiation therapy. Semin Radiat Oncol 2011;21(2):147–56.
15. Chu S, Karimi S, Peck KK, et al. Measurement of blood perfusion in spinal metastases with dynamic contrast-enhanced magnetic resonance imaging: evaluation of tumor response to radiation therapy. Spine 2013;38(22):E1418–24.
16. Morbée L, Chen M, Herregods N, et al. MRI-based synthetic CT of the lumbar spine: Geometric measurements for surgery planning in comparison with CT. Eur J Radiol 2021;144:109999.
17. Mastrogiacomo S, Dou W, Jansen JA, et al. Magnetic Resonance Imaging of Hard Tissues and Hard Tissue Engineered Bio-substitutes. Mol Imaging Biol 2019;21:1003–19.
18. Finkenstaedt T, Siriwananrangsun P, Achar S, et al. Ultrashort Time-to-Echo (UTE) 3-Tesla MRI for the Detection of Spondylolysis in Human Cadavers: Comparison with CT. Invest Radiol 2019; 54:32–8.
19. Afsahi AM, Lombardi AF, Wei Z, et al. High-Contrast Lumbar Spinal Bone Imaging Using a 3D Slab-Selective UTE Sequence. Front Endocrinol 2021; 12:800398.
20. Deininger-Czermak E, Villefort C, von Knebel Doeberitz N, et al. Comparison of MR Ultrashort Echo Time and Optimized 3D-Multiecho In-Phase Sequence to Computed Tomography for Assessment of the Osseous Craniocervical Junction. J Magn Reson Imaging 2021;53: 1029–39.
21. Böker SM, Adams LC, Bender YY, et al. Differentiation of Predominantly Osteoblastic and Osteolytic Spine Metastases by Using Susceptibility-weighted MRI. Radiology 2019;290:146–54.
22. Hong AL, Ispiryan M, Padalkar MV, et al. MRI-derived bone porosity index correlates to bone composition and mechanical stiffness. Bone Rep 2019;11:100213.
23. Figley CR, Yau D, Stroman PW. Attenuation of lower-thoracic, lumbar, and sacral spinal cord motion: implications for imaging human spinal cord structure and function. AJNR Am J Neuroradiol 2008;29(8): 1450–4.
24. Mikulis DJ, Wood ML, Zerdoner OA, et al. Oscillatory motion of the normal cervical spinal cord. Radiology 1994;192(1):117–21.
25. Tseng CL, Sussman MS, Atenafu EG, et al. Magnetic resonance imaging assessment of spinal cord and cauda equina motion in supine patients with spinal metastases planned for spine stereotactic body radiation therapy. Int J Radiat Oncol Biol Phys 2015; 91(5):995–1002.

26. Oztek MA, Mayr NA, Mossa-Basha M, et al. The Dancing Cord: Inherent Spinal Cord Motion and Its Effect on Cord Dose in Spine Stereotactic Body Radiation Therapy. Neurosurgery 2020; 87(6):1157–66.

27. Pfender N, Rosner J, Zipser CM, et al. Comparison of axial and sagittal spinal cord motion measurements in degenerative cervical myelopathy. J Neuroimaging 2022;32(6):1121–33.

28. Wolf K, Pfender N, Hupp M, et al. Spinal cord motion assessed by phase-contrast MRI - An intercenter pooled data analysis. Neuroimage Clin 2023;37: 103334.

29. MacLean MA, Touchette CJ, Georgiopoulos M, et al. AO Spine Knowledge Forum Tumor. Systemic considerations for the surgical treatment of spinal metastatic disease: a scoping literature review. Lancet Oncol 2022;23(7):e321–33.

Percutaneous Treatment of Spinal Metastases

Anderanik Tomasian, MD[a],*, Majid A. Khan, MD[b], Jack W. Jennings, MD, PhD[c]

KEYWORDS

• Spinal metastases • Thermal ablation • Vertebral augmentation • Thermal protection

KEY POINTS

- Percutaneous image-guided minimally invasive thermal ablation and vertebral augmentation are part of the robust armamentarium used by radiologists for the management of patients with spinal metastases.
- Thermal ablation is a safe and effective treatment in selected patients with vertebral metastases and is used to achieve pain palliation and local tumor control.
- Thermal protection is important to ensure procedure safety.

INTRODUCTION

Cancer is the second most common cause of death in the United States, and according to the American Cancer Society, approximately 1.9 million cases of new cancer diagnosis were expected in 2022, most of whom will develop metastases that in 40% of cases will involve the spine.[1] Skeletal-related events such as intractable pain due to direct bone involvement by tumor, pathologic fracture with or without mechanical instability, metastatic epidural spinal cord compression, and neurologic deficits often unfavorably influence patient functional independence and quality of life.[2,3]

When therapeutic decisions are made, the important limitations of external beam radiation therapy, the reference standard for pain palliation, and local tumor control of spinal metastases should be taken into consideration. Such limitations include the lack of optimal efficacy in offering adequate and timely pain palliation in up to 75% of patients, radiation-resistant tumors, and cumulative tolerance of the spinal cord, affecting further treatment of tumor progression or recurrence.[4,5] Surgical intervention, which is commonly reserved for patients with spinal instability or neurologic compromise, is limited by morbidity and typically

not entertained due to patient's frequent poor functional status. Moreover, spinal metastases may be inadequately responsive to systemic therapies such as chemotherapy, hormonal therapy, immunotherapy, radiopharmaceuticals, and bisphosphonates. In addition, the common side effects of opioids, and the often incomplete pain palliation, may render such medications inadequate for management of many patients.[6]

During the past several years, investigators have exploited minimally invasive percutaneous thermal ablation technologies, often combined with vertebral augmentation (VA), for management of vertebral metastases, with progressively robust data published in the recent literature supporting safety, efficacy, and durability of treatment.[7–29] Such interventions are performed to achieve pain palliation, local tumor control or cure, in conjunction with or supplemented by adjuvant radiation therapy, chemotherapy, or surgery. In consideration of the important benefits of these minimally invasive percutaneous techniques, the National Comprehensive Cancer Network (NCCN) and the American College of Radiology (ACR) have endorsed and incorporated thermal ablation and VA in the treatment guidelines of patients with spinal metastases.[30,31]

[a] University of California Irvine, 101 The City Drive South, Orange, CA, USA; [b] Thomas Jefferson University Hospital, 111 South 11th Street, Philadelphia, PA, USA; [c] Mallinckrodt Institute of Radiology, 510 South Kingshighway Boulevard, Saint Louis, MO, USA
* Corresponding author.
E-mail address: tomasian.andy@gmail.com

Neuroimag Clin N Am 33 (2023) 499–506
https://doi.org/10.1016/j.nic.2023.03.005
1052-5149/23/© 2023 Elsevier Inc. All rights reserved.

This article outlines the most recent advances in minimally invasive image-guided thermal ablation and VA and the role of radiologists in the management of patients with spinal metastases.

General Considerations, Treatment Goals, and Patient

Selection

A multidisciplinary approach is typically recommended to evaluate and select patients to undergo minimally invasive percutaneous thermal ablation for management of spinal metastases. The multidisciplinary team commonly includes radiologists, radiation oncologists, medical oncologists, and oncologic surgeons. Once a treatment consensus is reached, a pretreatment consultation is organized to reassess patient symptoms and perform a focused physical examination to reconfirm focal tenderness at the treatment target site and determine potential focal neurologic deficit.

The treatment goals of thermal ablation in patients with spinal metastases are to achieve pain palliation and local tumor control, along with cure (skeletal oligometastatic disease; fewer than five lesions).[7–29]

The primary indications for percutaneous thermal ablation, often performed with VA for pathologic fracture stabilization or prevention, include persistent pain or imaging evidence of tumor progression despite maximized radiation therapy, contraindications to radiation therapy, patient's lack of interest for radiation therapy, or insufficient treatment response to systemic therapies and analgesics/opioids. The main patient factors dictating eligibility for percutaneous thermal ablation for treatment of vertebral metastatic disease include pain, performance status, life expectancy, status of spinal stability and metastatic epidural spinal cord compression, and extent of visceral metastases.[7–9,11–19] Patient performance status is commonly determined using the validated and widely adopted Karnofsky Performance Status Scale.[32] The NCCN has recently adopted percutaneous thermal ablation into its guidelines for the management of bone metastases.[30] The latest NCCN guidelines for adult cancer pain (version 1.2022) indicate that thermal ablation may be considered for palliation of metastatic bone pain, in the absence of oncologic emergency, when chemotherapy is inadequate and radiation therapy is contraindicated or not desired by the patient.[30] The recently published ACR Appropriateness Criteria suggest the following guidelines for management of vertebral metastases[31]: Thermal ablation and VA may be appropriate for treatment of asymptomatic pathologic vertebral fracture with or without edema on MR imaging and are usually appropriate for treatment of pathologic vertebral fracture with severe and progressive pain. In addition, the ACR Appropriateness Criteria suggest that thermal ablation may be appropriate for treatment of pathologic vertebral fracture with spinal malalignment.[31]

Percutaneous thermal ablation, however, may be contraindicated in the context of spinal instability depending on severity. The severity of spinal instability is assessed using the spinal instability neoplastic score (SINS).[33] Surgical consultation for potential tumor resection/debulking and stabilization is typically considered for SINS of seven or higher.[33] Spinal metastases in the presence of central canal stenosis are commonly managed surgically[34]; however, in the absence of spinal cord compression, thermal ablation may be considered as an alternative approach in patients who are not surgical candidates. When central canal compromise is caused by tumor alone, thermal ablation may lead to arrest or retraction of epidural tumor.[9] However, thermal ablation will not alleviate symptoms in the presence of osseous retropulsion.

Thermal Ablation

Radiofrequency ablation

The latest generations of radiofrequency ablation (RFA) equipment, including navigational and bipolar electrodes, provide important advantages compared with traditional unipolar straight electrodes and are critical for patient safety and treatment outcomes, facilitating treatment of vertebral metastases in challenging anatomical locations.[7–10,14,17,27] Such advantages include electrode tip navigation, which can be articulated in different orientations through a single skin and osseous entry site, supporting treatment of challenging-to-access lesions along the posterior central vertebral body, achieving larger ablation zones, minimizing osseous weakening due to single bone access site, and improving efficiency. Additional advantages include precise real-time intraprocedural monitoring of ablation zone volume, made possible by built-in thermocouples along electrode shaft and bipolar technology eliminating the need for grounding pad placement and risk of electrode-related skin thermal injury[7–10,14,17,27] (Fig. 1). Furthermore, such RFA systems offer simultaneous bipedicular vertebral ablations resulting in larger, confluent, and coalescent ablation volumes.[9,27] Intact vertebral cortex serves as a relative barrier against undesired RF energy propagation which should be taken into account when spinal thermal ablation is considered as a therapeutic option.[35] Primary indications for utilization of RFA

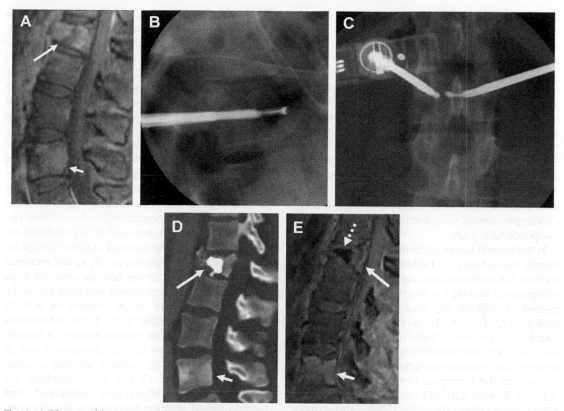

Fig. 1. A 32-year-old woman with metastatic breast cancer and painful L1 lesion. Sagittal T1-weighted contrast-enhanced MR imaging (A) shows enhancing bone marrow replacing metastatic lesion within the L1 vertebral body with pathologic fracture (A, long arrow). Note enhancing L4 vertebral body metastatic lesion which was not painful (A, short arrow). Radiofrequency ablation (RFA) was performed for pain palliation and local tumor control. Lateral and anterior-posterior fluoroscopic images during RFA (B, C) show bipedicular placement of two bipolar navigational electrodes within the anterior third of the L1 vertebral body, for treatment of clinical target volume with simultaneous ablations. Note the close proximity between the medial articulation of the right transpedicular electrode tip and the tip of the left transpedicular electrode to generate confluent coalescent ablation zone. Electrodes were subsequently retracted to treat the posterior aspect of the vertebral body and the pedicles (not shown). Thermal ablation was immediately followed by vertebral augmentation. Sagittal CT image (D) acquired 6 months following treatment shows cement within the treated vertebral body (D, long arrow). Note untreated L4 osteoblastic metastasis (D, short arrow). Sagittal T1-weighted contrast-enhanced MR imaging obtained 2 months following treatment (E) shows local tumor control with enhancing granulation tissue along the periphery of the ablation zone (E, long solid arrow). There is hypointense cement within the L1 vertebral body (E, dotted arrow). The untreated enhancing L4 vertebral body metastasis is again identified (E, short solid arrow).

for treatment of spinal metastases include the following: (1) primarily osteolytic or mixed osteolytic–osteoblastic metastases, (2) geographic spinal metastases with no or small extraosseous components, and (3) challenging-to-access lesions such as tumors along the posterior central vertebral body where access is feasible using navigational articulating electrodes (see Fig. 1). RFA is typically not considered as an option for treatment of densely osteoblastic metastases as the higher impedance of such tumors may render RFA ineffective.[36] In our practice, and in agreement with consensus recommendations from the International Spine

Radiosurgery Consortium, we recommend simultaneous bipedicular RFA for management of vertebral metastases to treat the entire clinical target volume (CTV) and achieve better local tumor control rates and more durable pain palliation[9,37] (see Fig. 1). CTV includes the gross tumor volume, plus the surrounding abnormal bone marrow signal intensity on MR imaging to account for microscopic tumor invasion, and the adjacent normal bone to account for subclinical tumor spread in marrow.[37] Such an approach translates into ablation of the entire vertebral body volume plus both pedicles, with two confluent, coalescent, and overlapping ablation zones in close proximity, minimizing convective cooling, risk of thermal injury, as well as tissue charring and impedance related issues (see **Fig. 1**).

The disadvantages of RFA include (1) computed-tomography (CT)-occult ablation zone, (2) convective cooling effect particularly with hypervascular metastases and cerebrospinal fluid as well as vertebral venous plexus flow, (3) relative ineffectiveness for treatment of densely osteoblastic tumors, (4) relative contraindication for use of monopolar electrodes in patients with metallic implants and pacemakers due to risk of skin thermal injury and pacemaker dysfunction, (5) intraprocedural pain, and (6) at times, increased periprocedural pain.[7–10,14,17,27]

In the largest series published to date on RFA of spinal metastases,[27] Tomasian and colleagues treated 266 metastatic lesions in 166 patients using navigational bipolar RF electrode system and reported statistically significant and durable pain palliation at 1-week, 1-month, 3-months, and 6-month posttreatment follow-up intervals with an overall local tumor control rate of 78.9%. The investigators documented procedural complications according to the Common Terminology Criteria for Adverse Events (CTCAE) classification system. A total complication rate of 3% (8/266) and a major complication rate of 0.4% (1/266) were reported.[27] The single major complication included lower extremity weakness, difficulty in urination, and lack of erection, as a result of spinal cord venous infarct. The seven minor complications included four cases of periprocedural transient radicular pain (CTCAE grade 2) requiring transforaminal steroid injections, one case of delayed secondary vertebral body fracture (CTCAE grade 2) requiring analgesics, and two cases of asymptomatic spinal cord edema on routine follow-up imaging (CTCAE grade 1).[27]

In a multicenter prospective study, Bagla and colleagues[8] treated 50 patients with spinal metastases (thoracolumbar spine) using RFA (69 ablations) and VA (96% of patients) and achieved statistically significant pain palliation and reduction in disability along with improvement in functional status and quality of life with no complications. In a multicenter prospective trial, Levy and colleagues[17] used RFA (combined with VA) for treatment of 100 patients with bone metastases, which included 87 patients with thoracolumbar lesions, and reported statistically significant pain palliation and improvement in quality of life at 6-month posttreatment interval with adverse effects rate of 3%.[17]

Cryoablation

During cryoablation, the initial freezing cycle (commonly 10 minutes) is immediately followed by a thawing phase (commonly 5–8 minutes), a second freezing cycle (commonly 10 minutes), and a second thawing phase (commonly 5–8 minutes).[11,12,14,28] Reliable cell death is achieved at the temperature of –40°C or lower.[38] As the hypoattenuating ice ball margin on CT corresponds to 0°C, ice ball extension beyond the tumor margins by at least 3–5 mm is recommended to ensure adequate ablation.[11,12,14,28] The recent generations of cryoprobes generate various distinct ablation zone volumes, which allow sculpting of desired ablation zones, particularly in close proximity to critical structures, whereas the relatively small gauge of such cryoprobes makes possible optimal applicator positioning.[11,12,14,28] The primary indications for the use of cryoablation for treatment of spinal metastases include (1) large tumors with complex geometry, (2) spinal metastases with large soft tissue components, (3) large tumors involving the posterior vertebral elements, (4) paravertebral soft tissue metastases, and (5) osteoblastic metastases (**Fig. 2**). The advantages of cryoablation include (1) visualization of hypoattenuating ice ball on CT, (2) concurrent use of several cryoprobes to achieve additive overlapping ablation zones, (3) less intraprocedural and immediate post-ablation pain compared with heating-based ablation techniques, and (4) availability of MR imaging-compatible cryoprobes. The disadvantages of cryoablation include (1) the often lack of discrete visualization of ice ball within osteoblastic metastases (and at times normal bone), (2) cost with use of several cryoprobes, (3) prolonged procedures in large tumors, and (4) delay in cementation to minimize interference with cement polymerization.

In a retrospective dual-center study, Cazzato and colleagues used cryoablation for treatment of 105 spinal metastases in 74 patients (combined with cementation in 72.4% of tumors).[28] The investigator reported statistically significant pain palliation at 1-day and 1-month post-procedural follow-up intervals as well as at the last available posttreatment follow-up (mean of 14.7 months, median of 6 months). A completely pain-free status was achieved at the last available follow-up in 53.1% of patients. The local tumor control rate was reported at 82.1% (mean follow-up of 25.9 months, median of 16.5 months).[28] The total complication rate was 8.5% (nine patients, including two major and seven minor complications).[28] Investigators treated 31 spinal metastases in 14 patients with cryoablation using thermoprotective techniques, and achieved 96.7% local tumor control, significant pain palliation, and decreased analgesics usage 1 week,

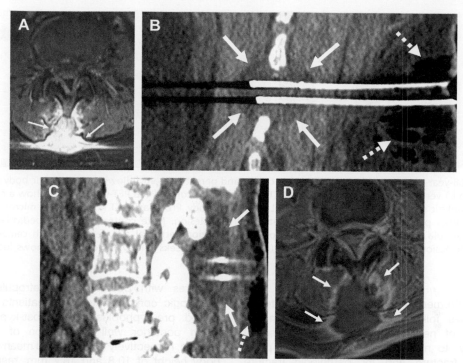

Fig. 2. A 63-year-old woman with metastatic lung squamous cell carcinoma with progressively enlarging and painful metastasis in the L2 spinous process despite radiation therapy. Axial T1-weighted contrast-enhanced MR imaging (A) shows destructive enhancing metastatic lesion in the spinous process of L2, extending to the paraspinal soft tissues (A, arrows). Cryoablation was performed for pain palliation and local tumor control. Oblique coronal and sagittal CT images during cryoablation (B, C) show placement of two cryoprobes within the lesion with hypoattenuating ice ball encompassing the lesion and extending to the surrounding tissues (B and C, solid arrows). Thermal protection of the skin was achieved with subcutaneous insufflation of carbon dioxide (B and C, dotted arrows). Axial T1-weighted contrast-enhanced MR imaging (D) obtained 2 months following cryoablation shows local tumor control with enhancing granulation tissue at the periphery of the ablation zone (D, arrows).

1 month, and 3 months after the procedure with no major complications.[11]

Microwave ablation

Although microwave ablation may be used for the treatment of spinal metastases that are not in close proximity to neural structures, this modality is most beneficial for treatment of spinal metastases with the following characteristics: (1) osteoblastic metastases and (2) large paraspinal tumors with complex geometry.

The advantages of microwave ablation include (1) less susceptibility to convective cooling and variable tumor tissue impedance, leading to more uniform and larger ablation volumes as well as improved efficiency compared with RFA, (2) the lack of need for grounding pad placement, (3) a concurrent use of multiple antennas to generate additive overlapping ablation volumes, (4) the minimal risk of back-heating phenomenon with recent generations of antennas, (e) and the lack of contra-indication in patients with metallic implants[13,19,26,29] (Fig. 3). The disadvantages of microwave ablation include

(1) largely CT-occult ablation zone, (2) less distinct ablation zone boundaries as compared with RFA and cryoablation, and (3) potential nontarget overheating due to rapid delivery of high-power output (up to 100 W) which should be considered when treating spinal metastases.[13,19,26,29]

In a single-center retrospective study, Chen and colleagues treated 140 spinal metastases in 91 patients with microwave ablation (combined with VA) and reported statistically significant pain palliation and reduction in opioid usage up to 6 months following treatment.[29] The investigators also documented decreased disability scores as well as a local tumor control rate of 94.8% at 6-month follow-up. Khan and colleagues successfully treated 102 spinal metastases (and myeloma) in 69 patients and reported statistically significant pain palliation at 2 to 4 week and 20 to 24-week post-procedural intervals as well as local tumor control rate of 97% at 20 to 24 weeks.[20] The investigators reported complications in two patients (S1 nerve thermal injury and skin burn).

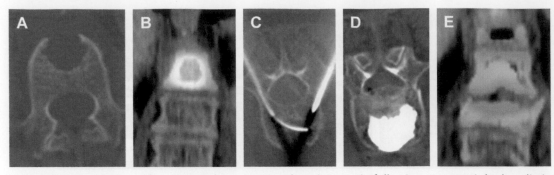

Fig. 3. A 68-year-old man with metastatic lung cancer and persistent pain following stereotactic body radiation therapy to L1 vertebral body metastasis. Axial CT image (A) and coronal F18 PET-CT image (B) show a hypermetabolic osteolytic metastasis within the anterior L1 vertebral body. Prone axial CT image during microwave ablation (C) shows placement of a curved antenna within the lesion. Note contralateral transpedicular cement delivery cannula. Prone axial CT image (D) shows post-ablation vertebral augmentation with cement within the treated lesion. Coronal F18 PET-CT image (E) obtained 12 weeks following treatment shows local tumor control.

Vertebral augmentation

VA is performed in most patients with vertebral metastases following thermal ablation, in the absence of neurologic compromise or spinal instability, to minimize the possibility of post-ablation fracture and for pathologic fracture stabilization[8–11,13,14,17,19,24,27,28] (see Fig. 1). VA may be performed as a stand-alone intervention for spinal metastases in patients with many osseous or visceral metastases.[21] The CAFÉ trial demonstrated that VA is effective as a stand-alone intervention to provide palliation by reducing pain and opioid usage while improving quality of life in a randomized controlled trial of 134 patients.[39] VA may not be indicated following thermal ablation of posterior vertebral elements only or of lower sacral spine segments. Investigators treated 72 vertebral pathologic fractures with epidural tumor involvement in 51 patients and achieved statistically significant pain palliation for 94%, 86%, and 92% of patients at 1-day, 1-month, and 1-year post-procedural intervals with a single case of cauda equina syndrome as a major complication.[22] Balloon kyphoplasty may improve the quality of tumor filling in spinal metastases. However, in cases with low risk of cement leakage, the use of balloon kyphoplasty may decrease cement interdigitation into the surrounding trabecular matrix, potentially compromising anchorage.[23] Kyphoplasty using a variety of spinal implants such as SpineJack, Kiva, vertebral body stents, and screw-assisted internal fixation has been used for management of vertebral pathologic compression fractures to restore vertebral body height, improve kyphosis, decrease osseous retropulsion, and improve central canal stenosis.[20] Venier and colleagues performed kyphoplasty with implants for 53 vertebral body fractures with posterior wall retropulsion (no neurologic compromise) in 51 patients and reported pre-kyphoplasty and post-kyphoplasty mean posterior wall retropulsion of 5.8 and 4.5 mm, respectively (P <.001) and mean vertebral body height of 10.8 and 16.7 mm, respectively (P< .001).[20] The investigators reported three new fractures at treated levels (follow-up of 1–36 months) for which no intervention was deemed necessary.[20]

Thermal protection

The important risk of undesired thermal injury to the spinal cord, spinal nerve roots, torso vital organs, and skin should be considered when planning percutaneous thermal ablation for spinal metastases. A variety of passive and active thermal protection techniques may be implemented to minimize the risk of thermal injury[7,9,11,14] (see Fig. 2).

Passive thermal protection techniques include evaluating patient biofeedback when ablating with the patient under conscious sedation (particularly heat-based ablations), real-time temperature monitoring by placement of thermocouples in the epidural space and neuroforamina, monitoring motor- and somatosensory-evoked potential amplitude and latency when ablating under general anesthesia, as well as conducting electro-stimulation of peripheral nerves for early detection of impending nerve injury.[7,9,11,14] Active thermal protection may be implemented prophylactically and is recommended when temperature reaches 45°C (heat) or 10°C (cold).[14,40] Active thermal protection is performed by thermal modification, displacement of the structure at risk, or thermal insulation using pneumo-dissection with carbon dioxide injection as well as hydro-dissection with injection of warm or cool liquid surrounding the at-risk structure. Skin thermal protection may be accomplished by precise assessment of ablation zone volume, active thermal protection of subcutaneous tissues, surface application of warm saline during cryoablation, and use of bipolar RF electrode systems.

SUMMARY

Recent developments in percutaneous minimally invasive thermal ablation and VA for the treatment of patients with spinal metastatic disease allow radiologists to provide safe, timely, and efficacious care with durable effects. The growing integration of such therapeutic approaches in clinical patient care will strengthen the radiologists' role in the care of such patients. The implementation of procedural safety techniques is critical to minimize potential adverse effects and improve patient outcomes.

DISCLOSURE

The authors have no commercial or financial conflicts of interest and no funding sources.

REFERENCES

1. Available at: https://www.cancer.org/content/dam/cancer-org/research/cancer-facts-and-statistics/annual-cancer-facts-and-figures/2022/2022-cancer-facts-and-figures.pdf. Accessed November 12, 2022.
2. Macedo F, Ladeira K, Pinho F, et al. Bone metastases: an overview. Oncol Rev 2017;11:321.
3. Urch C. The pathophysiology of cancer-induced bone pain: current understanding. Palliat Med 2004;18:267–74.
4. Strander H, Turesson I, Cavallin-Ståhl E. A systematic overview of radiation therapy effects in soft tissue sarcomas. Acta Oncol 2003;42:516–31.
5. van der Linden YM, Steenland E, van Houwelingen HC, et al. Dutch Bone Metastasis Study Group. Patients with a favourable prognosis are equally palliated with single and multiple fraction radiotherapy: results on survival in the Dutch Bone Metastasis Study. Radiother Oncol 2006;78:245–53.
6. Paice JA. Cancer pain management and the opioid crisis in America: How to preserve hard-earned gains in improving the quality of cancer pain management. Cancer 2018;124(12):2491–7.
7. Anchala PR, Irving WD, Hillen TJ, et al. Treatment of metastatic spinal lesions with a navigational bipolar radiofrequency ablation device: a multicenter retrospective study. Pain Physician 2014;17:317–27.
8. Bagla S, Sayed D, Smirniotopoulos J, et al. Multicenter prospective clinical series evaluating radiofrequency ablation in the treatment of painful spine metastases. Cardiovasc Intervent Radiol 2016;39:1289–97.
9. Tomasian A, Hillen TJ, Chang RO, et al. Simultaneous bipedicular radiofrequency ablation combined with vertebral augmentation for local tumor control of spinal metastases. AJNR Am J Neuroradiol 2018;39:1768–73.
10. Wallace AN, Tomasian A, Vaswani D, et al. Radiographic local control of spinal metastases with percutaneous radiofrequency ablation and vertebral augmentation. AJNR Am J Neuroradiol 2016;37:759–65.
11. Tomasian A, Wallace A, Northrup B, et al. Spine cryoablation:pain palliation and local tumor control for vertebral metastases. AJNR Am J Neuroradiol 2016;37:189–95.
12. Auloge P, Cazzato RL, Rousseau C, et al. Complications of percutaneous bone tumor cryoablation:a 10-year experience. Radiology 2019;291:521–8.
13. Khan MA, Deib G, Deldar B, et al. Efficacy and safety of percutaneous microwave ablation and cementoplasty in the treatment of painful spinal metastases and myeloma. AJNR Am J Neuroradiol 2018;39:1376–83.
14. Tomasian A, Gangi A, Wallace AN, et al. Percutaneous thermal ablation of spinal metastases: recent advances and review. AJR Am J Roentgenol 2018;210:142–52.
15. McMenomy BP, Kurup AN, Johnson GB, et al. Percutaneous cryoablation of musculoskeletal oligometastatic disease for complete remission. J Vasc Interv Radiol 2013;24:207–13.
16. Cazzato RL, Auloge P, De Marini P, et al. Percutaneous image-guided ablation of bone metastases: local tumor control in oligometastatic patients. Int J Hyperthermia 2018;35:493–9.
17. Levy J, Hopkins T, Morris J, et al. Radiofrequency Ablation for the Palliative Treatment of Bone Metastases:Outcomes from the Multicenter OsteoCool Tumor Ablation Post-Market Study (OPuS One Study) in 100 Patients. J Vasc Interv Radiol 2020;31(11):1745–52.
18. Cazzato RL, Palussière J, Auloge P, et al. Complications Following Percutaneous Image-guided Radiofrequency Ablation of Bone Tumors:A 10-year Dual-Center. Exp Radiol 2020;296(1):227–35.
19. Pusceddu C, Sotgia B, Fele RM, et al. Combined Microwave Ablation and Cementoplasty in Patients with Painful Bone Metastases at High Risk of Fracture. Cardiovasc Intervent Radiol 2016;39:74–80.
20. Venier A, Roccatagliata L, Isalberti M, et al. Armed Kyphoplasty:An Indirect Central Canal Decompression Technique in Burst Fractures. Am J Neuroradiol 2019;40(11):1965–72.
21. Wallace AN, Robinson CG, Meyer J, et al. The Metastatic Spine Disease Multidisciplinary Working Group algorithms. Oncol 2015;20:1205–15.

22. Saliou G, Kocheida EM, Lehmann P, et al. Percuta-neous vertebroplasty for pain management in malig-nant fractures of the spine with epidural involvement. Radiology 2010;254(3):882–90.

23. Dalton BE, Kohm AC, Miller LE, et al. Radiofre-quency targeted vertebral augmentation versus traditional balloon kyphoplasty:radiographic and morphologic outcomes of an ex vivo biomechanical pilot study. Clin Interv Aging 2012;7:525–31.

24. Wallace AN, Greenwood TJ, Jennings JW. Radiofre-quency ablation and vertebral augmentation for palliation of painful spinal metastases. J Neuro On-col 2015;124:111–8.

25. Tsoumakidou G, Koch G, Caudrelier J, et al. Image-guided spinal ablation: a review. Cardiovasc Inter-vent Radiol 2016;39:1229–38.

26. Kastler A, Alnassan H, Aubry S, et al. Microwave thermal ablation of spinal metastatic bone tumors. J Vasc Interv Radiol 2014;25:1470–5.

27. Tomasian A, Marlow J, Hillen TJ, et al. Complications of Percutaneous Radiofrequency Ablation of Spinal Osseous Metastases: An 8-Year Single-Center Experience. AJR Am J Roentgenol 2021;216(6): 1607–13.

28. Cazzato RL, Jennings JW, Autrusseau PA, et al. Percutaneous image-guided cryoablation of spinal metastases: over 10-year experience in two aca-demic centersEuropean. Radiology 2022;32: 4137–46.

29. Chen L, Hou G, Zhang K, et al. Percutaneous CT-Guided Microwave Ablation Combined with Verte-bral Augmentation for Treatment of Painful Spinal Metastases. AJNR Am J Neuroradiol 2022;43(3): 501–6.

30. National Comprehensive Cancer Network websi-te.NCCN clinical practice guidelines in oncology: adult cancer pain,version 1.2022. Available at: www. nccn.org. Accessed December 8, 2022.

31. Expert Panels on Neurological Imaging, Interven-tional Radiology, and Musculoskeletal Imaging, Shah LM, Jennings JW, Kirsch CFE, et al. ACR Appropriateness Criteria: management of vertebral compression fractures. J Am Coll Radiol 2018; 15(suppl 11):S347–64.

32. Schag CC, Heinrich RL, Ganz PA. Karnofsky perfor-mance status revisited:reliability,validity, and guide-lines. J Clin Oncol 1984;2:187–93.

33. Fisher CG, DiPaola CP, Ryken TC, et al. A novel clas-sification system for spinal instability in neoplastic disease:an evidence-based approach and expert consensus from the Spine Oncology Study Group. Spin (Phila Pa 1976) 2010;35:E1221–9.

34. Patchell RA, Tibbs PA, Regine WF, et al. Direct de-compressive surgical resection in the treatment of spinal cord compression caused by metastatic can-cer:a randomised trial. Lancet 2005;366:643–8.

35. Dupuy DE, Hong R, Oliver B, et al. Radiofrequency ablation of spinal tumors: temperature distribution in the spinal canal. AJR Am J Roentgenol 2000; 175:1263–6.

36. Singh S, Saha S. Electrical properties of bone:a re-view. Clin Orthop Relat Res 1984;186:249–71.

37. Cox BW, Spratt DE, Lovelock M, et al. International Spine Radiosurgery Consortium consensus guide-lines for target volume definition in spinal stereotac-tic radiosurgery. Int J Radiat Oncol Biol Phys 2012; 83:e597–605.

38. Weld KJ, Landman J. Comparison of cryoablation,-radiofrequency ablation and high-intensity focused ultrasound for treating small renal tumours. BJU Int 2005;96:1224–9.

39. Berenson J, Pflugmacher R, Jarzem P, et al. Cancer Patient Fracture Evaluation (CAFE) Investigators. Balloon kyphoplasty versus non-surgical fracture management for treatment of painful vertebral body compression fractures in patients with cancer: a multicentre, randomised controlled trial. Lancet Oncol 2011;12(3):225–35.

40. Buy X, Tok CH, Szwarc D, et al. Thermal protection during percutaneous thermal ablation procedures: interest of carbon dioxide dissection and tempera-ture monitoring. Cardiovasc Intervent Radiol 2009; 32:529–34.

The Role of 3D Printing in Treatment Planning of Spine and Sacral Tumors

Jonathan M. Morris, MD[a],*, Adam Wentworth, MS[b],
Matthew T. Houdek, MD[c], S. Mohammed Karim, MD[c],
Michelle J. Clarke, MD[d], David J. Daniels, MD, PhD[d], Peter S. Rose, MD[c]

KEYWORDS

- 3D printing • Spine • Spine tumor • Spine metastasis • Surgical planning • Spine navigation
- Osteotomy guide • Patient-specific instrument

KEY POINTS

- Three-dimensional (3D) printing is an additive technology that allows the creation of life size patient-specific anatomic and pathologic models from multimodality cross-sectional data
- 3D-printed models provide a deeper understanding of critical anatomic relationships for the surgeon, referring clinician, and patient, which improves patient-specific preoperative planning, simulation, and education.
- Virtual surgical planning and 3D-printed custom osteotomy guides aid in obtaining negative margins, limiting normal tissue resection, and improving confidence in the resection of complex tumors in the spine and sacrum.
- 3D printing opens the possibilities of manufacturing complex geometries, such as lattice structures in titanium, for improved implant design and custom, one of a kind patient matched implants.

INTRODUCTION

Three-dimensional (3D) printing is a rapidly evolving technology that has revolutionized several industries, including medicine and surgery. This expansion in medicine has been facilitated by the convergence of advancements in manufacturing technologies, cross-sectional imaging, the availability of user-friendly medical 3D computer-aided design (CAD) software, and growing clinical indications. The ability to create precise, patient-specific anatomic and pathologic models has advanced surgical preoperative planning, intraoperative decision-making, education, and custom as well as off-the-shelf 3D-printed implant design. In particular, 3D printing has emerged as a promising tool in spine and sacral surgery. Coupled with new surgical techniques, 3D printing has aided

in the surgical correction of increasing complex spine deformities, improved outcomes during complex oncologic resections, and allowed the manufacturing of custom implants. In this review, we discuss the advancements in 3D printing technology, its applications in oncologic surgery of the spine and sacrum, and highlight the challenges and opportunities associated with adopting this technology at the point of care.

THREE-DIMENSIONAL PRINTING/ADDITIVE MANUFACTURING
Technology

A detailed discussion of each 3D printing technology, along with its advantages, disadvantages, and associated post-processing equipment, is beyond the scope of this review. However, a brief

[a] Division of Neuroradiology, Department of Radiology, Anatomic Modeling Unit, Biomedical and Scientific Visualization, Mayo Clinic, 200 1st Street, Southwest, Rochester, MN, 55905, USA; [b] Department of Radiology, Anatomic Modeling Unit, Mayo Clinic, Rochester, MN, USA; [c] Division of Orthopedic Oncology, Orthopedic Surgery, Mayo Clinic, Rochester, MN, USA; [d] Department of Neurosurgery, Mayo Clinic, Rochester, MN, USA
* Corresponding author.
E-mail address: morris.jonathan@mayo.edu

Neuroimag Clin N Am 33 (2023) 507–529
https://doi.org/10.1016/j.nic.2023.05.001

introduction to the manufacturing capabilities and common post-processing steps of the 7 most common 3D printing technologies in medicine has been summarized in Table 1. 3D printing is an umbrella term used to represent the 7 American Society for Testing and Materials International standards.[1] Each of these 7 standards is also an umbrella category, each with unique printing technologies, varied materials, and advantages and disadvantages for different medical uses. It is necessary to have a working knowledge of these technologies and their capabilities if an institution is considering setting up a point of care manufacturing facility.

Manufacturing Workflow

Imaging

Several steps are involved in making 3D-printed patient-specific models or custom medical devices (Fig. 1). The first is setting up an ordering system locally through your institution's electronic medical record (EMR) or using a HIPPA compliant data transfer agreement with an external vendor. This order triggers the appropriate imaging protocol for 3D printing, which in some cases, such as the spine and sacrum, differs from the protocol for diagnosis. In our institution, we have set up several protocols related to 3D printing that are available to the technologist, fulfilling the order at one of several different locations and using computed tomography (CT) or magnetic resonance imaging (MRI) scanners. For example, tumors involving the sacrum or retroperitoneum and invading into the spine are protocoled using a thin section (0.75 mm) CT angiogram (CTA), CT venogram, 3 minute delayed CT urogram (CTU), as well as a 10 minute delayed CTU with soft tissue reconstruction algorithms because it is helpful to have all of the vascular structures, the ureters, the bladder, the bone, and the tumor co-registered into one model. Because each anatomic structure must be segmented as separate objects in CAD software to be printed in different colors/materials, it is important to have the patient immobilized between scans, perform a tight bolus during CTA to avoid venous contamination, and ensure that the urographic phase is captured (see Fig. 1). For CT of the spine or cervical through the thoracic spine, it is important to scan the range in one pass and not move the arms up or down, as would be typical for diagnostic imaging.

Segmentation

DICOM images are then transferred to software that is capable of segmentation and co-registration of multiphase CT and co-registration of CT and MRI. Currently, it is recommended, per the FDA guidance

document, that clinical use of 3D printing should utilize 510(k)-approved software.[2] Examples include Mimics (Materialise, Leuven, Belgium) and DICOM 2 Print (D2P, 3D Systems, Rock Hill, SC). The images then undergo segmentation, which is the process of marking an anatomic region of interest (ROI) or target regions of similar properties on imaging and dividing it into anatomical structures.[3,4] Segmentation can be performed manually, using automated/semiautomated rule-based techniques, machine learned algorithms, or a combination of the three.[5–16] The ROIs are interpolated from the imaging to generate a surface-based 3D model, which is then exported into a medical CAD program.

Computer-aided design and virtual surgical planning

Following segmentation, the surface-based 3D anatomic model is converted to a CAD file format, most commonly the stereolithography (STL) format. An STL file represents and fits the 3D surface of the model as a triangular mesh (see Fig. 1F).[17] Multiple other CAD file formats, such as Virtual Reality Modeling Language (VRML/WRL), Wavefront OBJ (OBJ), Additive Manufacturing File (AMF), and 3D Manufacturing Format (3MF), can also be used throughout the 3D printing workflow, depending on the need for color and texture mapping.[18] In the CAD program, the user can make minor modifications such as restricting the ROI to be printed, placing cylinders to hold anatomic parts together, cutting the model and placing magnet casings to view internal components, hollowing and smoothing, and repairing the mesh (Fig. 2). Alternatively, major modifications occur in this step, such as mirror imaging to make a perfected anatomy, virtual removal of tumors, medical device sizing and virtual placement, and virtual surgical planning[19] (see Fig. 2). Finally, a unique patient identification label is placed on each model digitally before exporting to print.

Three-dimensional printing

Beginning as one technology in the 1980s,[20–22] the field has exponentially advanced to now include many technologies and capabilities. When selecting a 3D printing modality for clinical applications, multiple considerations must be taken regarding the need for color, material properties, transparency, biocompatibility, sterilization, accuracy levels, turnaround time, and the cost of capital equipment/consumables.[23,24] Once a production plan is decided upon, the CAD-modified model or patient-specific device is exported as a CAD file format compatible with the 3D printer (eg, STL, VRML/WRL, OBJ/MTL, AMF, and 3MF). Files

Table 1
Summary of 3D printing technologies

Additive Manufacturing Technology	Process Description	Technologies	Common Materials	Medical Uses	Pros	Cons
Vat Photopolymerization	Vat polymerization is a 3D printing process that selectively cures a liquid resin layer-by-layer using a light source, such as a UV laser or projector.	Stereolithography Digital light processing	Photopolymer (Thermoset) resins Biocompatible photopolymer resins	Single color anatomic models, Clear models, Surgical osteotomy guides, small jigs and fixtures, injection molding	1. High accuracy and resolution 2. Complex parts 3. Smooth surface finish 4. Cost effective 5. Widely available 6. Fastest print times	1. No color 2. Single material 3. Affected by UV light after the print 4. Relatively brittle 5. Multistep post-processing
Material Extrusion	Material filaments are passed through a heated nozzle, similar to a hot glue gun, and deposited on a platform that moves up and down vertically after each new layer is deposited	Fuse deposition modeling Fused filament fabrication	Thermoplastic polymers that come in filaments (eg, PLA, ABS, TPU)	Single color anatomic models, jigs and fixtures, prosthetic attachments	1. Inexpensive 2. Widely available 3. Low cost 4. Good structural properties 5. Ease of post-processing	1. Lower accuracy 2. Rough finish 3. Slow 4. Prone to error
Binder Jetting	Liquid binder is selectively deposited through inkjet nozzles, similar to 2D printers, along the x and y axes onto a powder bed, one layer at a time.	Binder jetting (BJ)	Gypsum, metals, sand, and ceramics that come in powder.	Multicolor anatomic models, Osseous simulation models, Molds, sand casting	1. Low Cost 2. Full Color 3. No support material 4. Can be infiltrated with multiple materials 5. Fast print times 6. Uses build volume (bin stacking)	1. Fragile 2. Green parts have poor mechanical properties and are brittle 3. Limited material selection

(continued on next page)

Table 1
(*continued*)

Additive Manufacturing Technology	Process Description	Technologies	Common Materials	Medical Uses	Pros	Cons
Material Jetting	Similar to 2D printers, a printhead dispenses droplets of a photosensitive material that solidifies under ultraviolet (UV) light, building a part layer-by-layer.	Material jetting (MJ) Drop on demand (DOD)	Thermoset photopolymer (acrylics) in liquid form. Biocompatible photopolymer	Clear, flexible, and full color anatomic models, Photo realistic models, Sterilizable guides, dental appliances	1. High accuracy and resolution 2. Smooth surface finish 3. Photo realistic color, clear, flexible multi-material all in one print 4. Wide range of materials 5. Medical polymers are sterilizable	1. Expensive 2. Long print times 3. Ultrasonic baths and pressurized nozzles needed for support removal 4. Fragile parts 5. Mechanic properties degrade over time
Powder Bed Fusion	Uses a laser or electron beam to melt and fuse material powders together layer by layer. Electron beam melting (EBM), methods require a vacuum. Selective heat sintering (SHS) differs by using a heated thermal print head to fuse powder material.	Selective laser sintering Direct metal laser sintering SHS Selective laser melting Electron beam melting	Thermoplastics such as polyamide (nylon) 11 and 12, aluminum, carbon filled aluminum, glass filled nylon	Titanium implants (eg, spine cages, orthopedic implant, CMF plates, dental, and custom titanium lattice structures), anatomic model, sterilizable guides, molds	1. No support material 2. Good isotropic mechanical properties (not fragile) 3. Ability to reuse un-sintered powder 4. Custom titanium implants 5. Custom metal lattice structures 6. Can be colored postproduction	1. Long time to print and let cool 2. Prone to warping and shrinkage 3. Grainy surface finish 4. Expensive 5. Only available in in-dustrial settings 6. Metal requires mul-tiple expensive post-processing

Sheet Lamination	Laminated object manufacturing (LOM) UAM Plastic sheet lamination (PSL)	Laminated object manufacturing (LOM) prints color on paper, which is then cut and bonded together with an adhesive. Ultrasonic additive manufacturing (UAM) uses sheets or ribbons of metal welded together. The final shape achieved by CNC machining or laser cutting	Paper, most polymers, plastics, Sheet metals, carbon fiber combined with thermoplastics, PEEK	Visual anatomic models	1. Speed 2. Low cost 3. Color models 4. Ease of handling materials 5. Fast 6. Multiple materials possible 7. No support structures	1. Limited material chooses 2. Low strength 3. Part Resolution limited by thickness of sheet 4. Cannot make hollow parts 5. Bonding strength limits long term use
Direct Energy Deposition	Electron beam additive manufacturing Laser deposition welding Direct metal deposition Laser engineered net shaping	Melting materials, either powders or wire sources, and depositing them on the workpiece, layer by layer. A nozzle mounted on a multi-axis (5) arm inside a closed frame, which deposits melted material onto the workpiece surface, where it solidifies.	Metals: Titanium and titanium alloys, inconel, tantalum, tungsten, niobium, stainless steel, and aluminum	No significant role in medical applications	1. Large parts 2. Repair metal parts	1. Large industrial machines 2. Expensive 3. Low resolution 4. Poor surface quality

Adapted from Guttridge C, Shannon A, O'Sullivan A, et al. Biocompatible 3D printing resins for medical applications: A review of marketed intended use, biocompatibility certification, and post-processing guidance. Annals of 3D Printed Medicine, Volume 5. 2022. 100044.

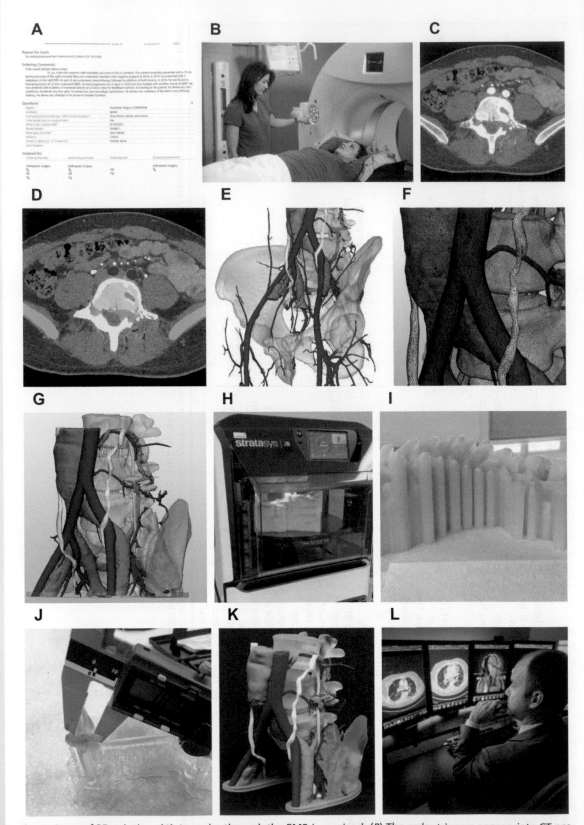

Fig. 1. Steps of 3D printing. (*A*) An order through the EMR is received. (*B*) The order triggers appropriate CT protocol on one of several scanners. (*C*) 3 phase CTA, CTV, CTU, and delayed CTU of patient with metastatic leiomyosarcoma metastasis in L5. (*D*) Segmentation of desired structures. (*E*) 3D surface model exported to a medical CAD

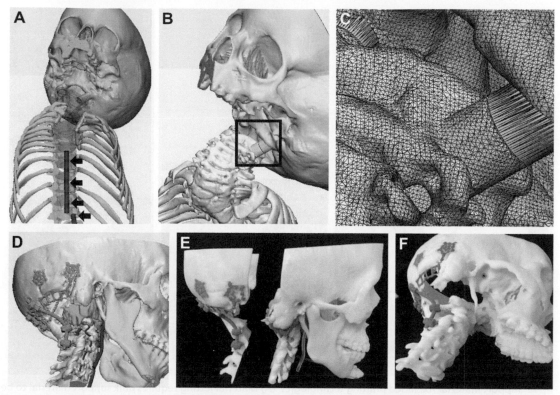

Fig. 2. Minor and major modifications to 3D-printed models. (*A*) A transparent CAD model demonstrates cylinders that need to be placed inside the model to provide structural stability when manufactured, particularly in pediatric cases where full ossification centers have not formed yet. Black arrows. (*B, C*) Magnet housings (*black box*) designed in CAD are placed at the craniocervical junction and boolean unioned with the anatomy in order to manufacture the skull separate from the spine so that the 2 parts are removable from each other. (*D*) 3D OBJ CAD model of recurrent high-grade meningioma (green), skull, mandible, arteries, and hardware involving the craniocervical junction with previous fusion. (*E*) A designed curved cut plane with magnet casings allows the posterior patient matched 3D-printed anatomy to be removed, allowing a full view of the tumor. (*F*) Virtual tumor removal was performed in CAD and then 3D-printed using material jetting to demonstrate the size of the defect once the tumor was removed for postoperative reconstruction planning.

are then inputted into build processing or slicing software and then printed layer by layer. Because 3D printers have been shown to have interprinter reliability issues and can have single printer build failures, a robust quality control system is needed for accurate manufacturing. A detailed introduction to a recommended quality control system for 3D printers and their operation can be found in other publications.[25]

Post-processing
After the 3D printing is complete, support material needs to be removed depending on the technology, and the product is cleaned of residual manufacturing

materials (Fig. 3). The type and extent of cleaning depend on the 3D printing technology used to manufacture the model or device. The 3D printer's original equipment manufacturer has instructions for cleaning and post-processing, and these recommendations must be followed during this step. Removing struts or residual materials could cause incidental harm or damage to the final anatomical model or devices and must be performed cautiously. Further post-processing steps include infiltration of liquids into powder-based models, photobleaching and buffing of clear models, and in the case of metal implant 3D printing, heat treatments (HIPPING or annealing) and screw threading are performed.

---

program. (*F, G*) CAD model is modified, fixed, and smoothed; ROI to be printed is chosen, and colors are assigned. (*H*) The model is resliced and printed layer by layer on one of several 3D printers. (*I*) Post-processing to remove support material and any other necessary steps. (*J*) Quality control steps are performed. (*K*) 3D-printed model is delivered to the ordering team. (*L*) Model is dictated and billed.

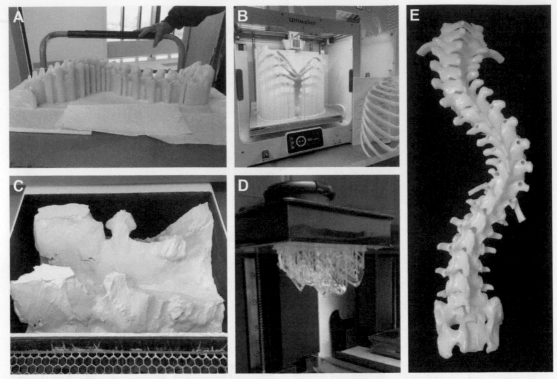

Fig. 3. Support material for varied printing technologies. (*A*) Material jetting requires bulk support material to be removed by hand; the print is then soaked in a lye bath, and then water blasted if needed, making small, fragile parts difficult to post process. (*B*) Material extrusion uses several types of support material, but most are water soluble making post less complicated. (*C*) Powder-based 3D printing technologies (powder bed fusion, binder jetting) use the unfused powder as support material, which is then reclaimed automatically, broken apart by hand, or vacuumed away to reveal the underlying part. (*D*) Vat photopolymerization (SLA, DLP) parts use scaffolds as support materials that have to be manually removed after alcohol soaking and photocuring. (*E*) Final part, 3D-printed spine from A, after removal of support material.

Point of care manufacturing

Traditional medical manufacturing remains the gold standard for most hospital systems and will likely remain so for most products a surgeon encounters. However, point-of-care manufacturing (POCM) using 3D printing is a rapidly growing field that offers numerous benefits for patients, radiologists, and surgeons. POCM involves the production of diagnostic anatomic models, sterilizable osteotomy guides, custom surgical instruments, pedicle screw trajectory guides, and implants at the point of care rather than in a centralized, traditional manufacturing facility. At our institution, we have a centralized POCM facility in the hospital, specifically in the radiology department, that serves all surgical subspecialties. This has allowed us to construct a specialized facility and centralize not only the hardware and software but all of the subspecialty skill sets, including radiologists, engineers, health care technology maintenance personnel, segmenters, artists, extended reality engineers, and administrative support staff.[15]

Over the last 17 years, we have found that this approach allows the greatest cross-pollination of ideas, improved collaboration, faster production times, and reduced costs compared with traditional manufacturing methods.

In addition to the broad benefits of POCM in medicine, this approach has specific advantages for spine and sacral surgery, particularly in tumor planning and resection. Traditionally, a surgeon will send anonymized DICOM images through a cloud-based HIPPA-compliant transfer mechanism to a medical device company, which will perform segmentation. In some instances, the device company will attempt to segment the tumor along with other structures and then return the file to the surgeon for approval. In this case, neither party has subspecialty expertise to define the boundaries of a metastasis or a primary bone tumor if local control is the goal. Having a subspecialist radiologist who understands imaging limitations and tumor infiltration using all available studies is crucial, particularly in the resection of

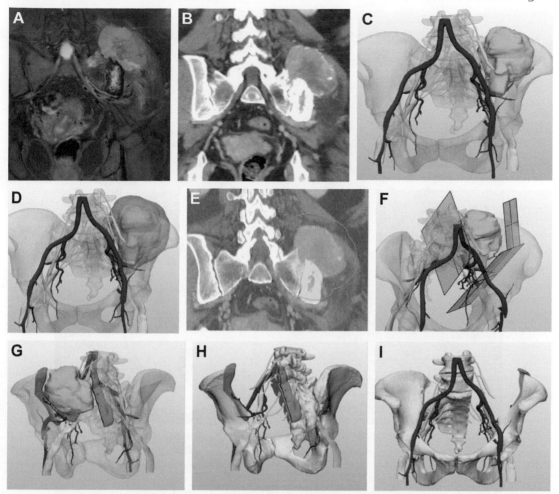

Fig. 4. Segmentation of tumor margins in a 43 year old male with an epithelioid hemangioendothelioma of the left iliac bone invading the sacrum. (*A, B*) A fat saturated coronal T2WI and coronal CT scan demonstrate a 7.7 cm aggressive mass in the left iliac bone infiltrating the lateral sacrum (*C*). A 3D CAD model demonstrates the tumor and adjacent critical anatomy, segmented by a board certified radiologist with subspecialty training in musculoskeletal bone tumors. (*D*) 1.5 cm margin is produced in medical CAD software from the original segmentation. (*E*) The new tumor volume is copied back to the original segmented data to determine if the margin can be obtained while preserving the lumbosacral plexus. (*F*) Through a collaborative relationship with the referring surgeon at the point of care, cut planes are designed. (*G*) 3D-printed patient matched cutting guides are designed to be screwed onto the underlying bone. (*H, I*) 3D CAD model with virtually removed tumor and bone for reconstruction planning.

primary bone tumors, as opposed to separation surgery. Although advances in automated segmentation algorithms for bone tumors[26–29] have occurred, they are not widely or commercially available. Sometimes, the algorithm or a trained segmenter can begin the process. However, at our institution, all tumor cases, including those involving the spine and sacrum, undergo hand segmentation by the radiologist, assuring accurate tumor margins and, in some cases, planning an additional 2 cm negative margin for guided resection if the anatomy allows for it (Fig. 4). This is a significant advantage for POCM because it allows faster, more accurate virtual surgical planning, changes the surgical approach 5% to 15% of the

time depending on the specialty, and if needed, provides an accurate plan for patient-specific custom medical device creation either locally or with a traditional manufacturer.

THREE-DIMENSIONAL PRINTED ANATOMIC AND PATHOLOGIC MODELS: SPINE AND SACRAL TUMORS
Patient-Specific Three-Dimensional Printed Diagnostic Models for Tumors of the Spine and Sacrum

Since the advent of CT and MRI, our ability to peer inside the body using cross-sectional data has widely expanded our diagnostic and interventional

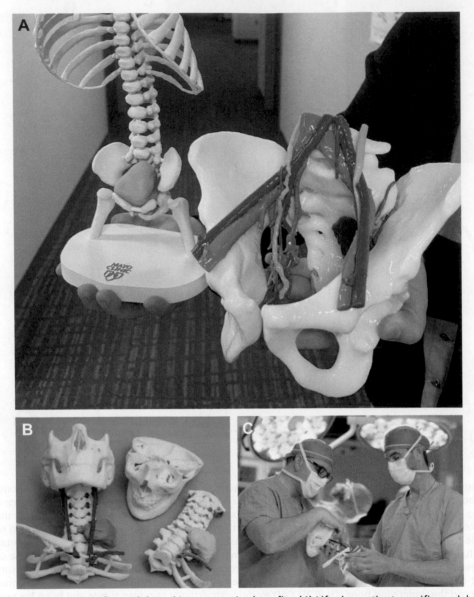

Fig. 5. Life size patient-specific models and intraoperative benefits. (*A*) Life size patient-specific models of an infant with prostatic rhabdomyosarcoma infiltrating the presacral space held next to an adult with a lateral sacral chondrosarcoma demonstrate the dramatic size differences not typically appreciated on radiology viewing systems. (*B*) 3D-printed model of a 12 year old female with an aneurysmal bone cyst at C6 with epidural extension, compressive myelopathy, and paraspinal extension. (*C*) Intraoperative collaboration between surgeons using the model as a common vehicle of communication to discuss the approach and steps of the procedure.

capabilities. Modern CT has progressed to perform high-speed acquisition of thin slice volumetric data, allowing the ability to perform an array of 3D post-processing techniques, including maximal intensity projections, minimum intensity projections, and finally, 3D surface shaded volume rendering (SS-VRT).[30] These 3D visualization techniques, in turn, led to improved diagnostic understanding of complex anatomy and pathology.[31–34] 3D representations have several limitations,

including a lack of life size scale when viewing them and utilizing only visual perception without the added benefits of haptic perception. Understanding 3D data from cross-sectional imaging can be improved with greater exposure, but creating a 3D representative object from 2D sequential slices within the mind is extremely complex.[35–38] There remains a significant challenge in translating these digital 3D representations on a screen to what a surgeon sees in the operative room, either in open or minimally invasive procedures. Additionally, over the last decade, there has been an exponential increase in the number of images per study and imaging modalities per patient, leaving the surgeon to evaluate an ever-increasing amount of data to construct complex patient-specific 3D anatomic and pathologic relationships mentally.[39] 3D printing life size patient matched models, particularly of the spine and sacrum, in the system described above aids in the surgeons' ability to understand patient-specific anatomy and pathology visually and tangibly preoperatively and intraoperatively[40–42] (**Fig. 5**). To guide the use of 3D-printed preoperative diagnostic anatomic and pathologic models in medicine, the Radiological Society of North America Special Interest Group on 3D Printing published guidelines on clinical appropriateness based on a comprehensive review of the literature.[43] There is significant evidence that it is appropriate for preoperative planning of complex bone and soft tissue neoplasms and notably indicated for complex spine and sacral oncologic cases, given the implicit complexity of the anatomy, the increased potential for complications, and the need for careful preoperative surgical planning with respect to critical surrounding structures. This is crucial when planning resection of primary bone tumors involving the spine, where long-term disease-free survival depends on en bloc tumor removal with negative margins[44–47] and even more crucial in the cervical spine and sacrum, where critical nerves and the vertebral

arteries can cause significant morbidity or limit en bloc resectability[48–51] (**Fig. 6**).

Benefits of 3D-printed preoperative patient-specific models[52–62]

- Detailed preoperative planning and improved confidence in the surgical intervention.
- Improved anatomic relationships to critical neural and neurovascular structures.
- Increased accuracy and efficiency in implant and screw positioning.
- Improved accuracy of osteotomy and vertebrectomy.
- Decreased reference to other imaging resources intraoperatively.
- 5% to 10% change in surgical approach (eg, reduced number of levels instrumented and intraoperative positioning)
- Decreased operative time.
- Feasibility of large tumor resections and multi-level vertebrectomy
- Improved pedicle screw trajectory planning in severe deformities
- Guiding fibula, iliac crest, or femur osseous grafts (**Fig. 7**)
- Improved understanding of tumor recurrence or reconstruction failure in previously operated patients needing a second or third operation
- Haptic perception of complex anatomy (**Fig. 8**)
- Improved intraoperative navigation confidence when a model is present

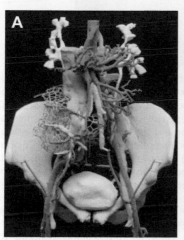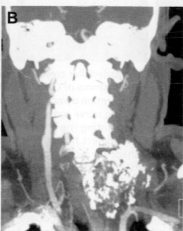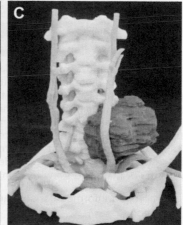

Fig. 6. Complexity of en bloc resection of primary tumors involving the sacrum and cervical spine. (*A*) 3D-printed model of an L5 chondrosarcoma extending into the sacrum and encasing the iliac vasculature, making multidisciplinary resection complicated. (*B*) Coronal CTA demonstrates an osteosarcoma involving C5–C7 and encasing the vertebral artery. (*C*) 3D-printed model of the tumor, bone, and vasculature with a detachable clavicle through magnetic casings. A conversation with the patient to discuss the treatment goals of a potential local cure and a four-quarter amputation with vertebral artery sacrifice versus subtotal resection followed by radiation is aided by the 3D-printed model.

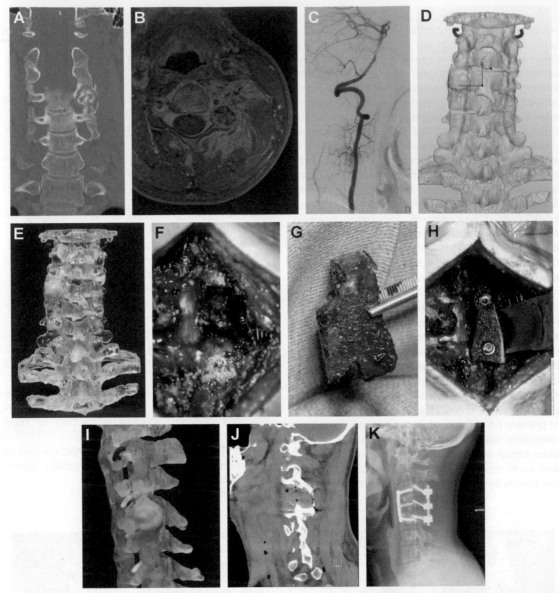

Fig. 7. En bloc removal of C4 osteoblastoma with guided iliac crest autograft. (*A*, *B*) Coronal CT scan and fat satu-rated post gadolinium T1WI demonstrate an osteoblastoma of C4 with marked surrounding edema. (*C*) An angio-gram to perform a balloon occlusion test and embolization demonstrates increased vascularity of the mass. (*D*) 3D CAD file of the model, including bone, tumor, exiting nerve roots, and arteries, was created from the segmenta-tion. (*E*) Material jetting 3D-printed model allows printing the bone in clear and the tumor, nerves, and vascula-ture in color. (*F*) Intraoperative photograph of the defect from the en bloc reception of the tumor. (*G*) Custom shaped iliac crest bone graft was formed in a T shape for reconstruction. (*H*) Autograft in place, filling the defect. (*I*) Sagittal view of a 3D-printed model. (*J*) Sagittal postoperative CT scan showing the T shaped graft in position. (*K*) Anterior plate and screw fixation, C3/4 and C4/5 discectomy, and posterior screw and rod fixation.

- Improved informed consent and patient edu-cation (Fig. 9)
- Improved patient-specific trainee education
- Steepening of the preoperative planning learning curve

Limitations, Barriers, and Billing

There are some existing barriers to offering POCM at each institution. First is the cost of the infrastructure and software, as well as the cost of the models, which can range from $100.00 for sin-gle color fuse deposition modeling models to $2000.00 for multicolor, multi-material, and clear material jetting models. This is typically offset by the reduction in operative times, which can range from $80.00 to $100.00 per minute in the United States, as well as the decrease in postoperative complications and morbidity by improved surgical

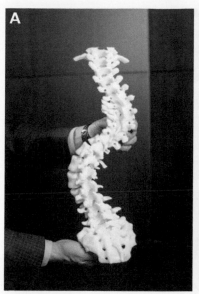
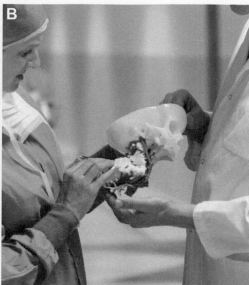

Fig. 8. Haptic perception benefits of 3D-printed models of the spine. (*A*) 3D-printed model of complex thoracolumbar scoliosis is better understood by holding the physical model. Giving the surgeon a complete view of the patient's spine with pedicle screw trajectories preplanned. (*B*) Team members discuss complex spine cases by physically interacting with a life size digital twin of the patient, driving deeper understanding through touch and visual perception.

planning. Additionally, at our institution, we maintain a digital thread of the medical model/guide (starting with a medical order through the EMR and ultimately ending in a dictation), which triggers the billing mechanisms of the model and guides to third party payers, further offsetting the cost. In July 2019, Category III Current Procedural Terminology Codes were approved and published by the American Medical Association, including patient-specific anatomic models (0559T and 0560T) and surgical guides (0561T and 0562T).[63,64] With an increasing number of PCOM facilities, the above benefits, and category III billing codes, the market has also started to provide these services to hospitals that require patient-specific models but do not want to invest in an on-premises solution. These include RICOH (Tokyo, Japan), Axial 3D (Belfast, Ireland), Stratasys (Eden Prairie, MN), 3D life prints (West Derby, England), and Osteo 3D (Andover, Massachusetts), to name a few. Other barriers include the need for qualified POCM engineers, segmenters, and radiologists and the lack of commercially available medical device production systems, leaving the end user to deploy their own quality control system, which they may not be qualified to deploy. There are attempts to improve the availability of staff with knowledge of 3D printing, anatomy, pathology, radiology, medical device design, and good manufacturing principles by coordinated efforts from the RSNA 3D Special Interest Group,

the Society of Manufacturing Engineering, and the American Society of Manufacturing Engineering for workforce development in this specialty.[65]

THREE-DIMENSIONAL PRINTED PEDICLE SCREW TRAJECTORY AND CUSTOM OSTEOTOMY GUIDES
Three-Dimensional Printed Pedicle Screw Trajectory Guides

Surgical treatment of tumors involving the spine, either for metastatic disease or primary bone tumors, typically undergoes one of 2 strategies: (1) Palliative surgery with cord decompression and follow-up radiation therapy or cord separation surgery or (2) curative surgery with en bloc resection of the tumor or for resection of more benign lesions. Both require spine immobilization and stabilization to enhance spinal fusion using posterior pedicle screw fixation. Originally, pedicle screws were placed using a freehand technique[66] but assisted techniques using fluoroscopy and intraoperative CT navigation were developed.[67–71] More recently, minimally invasive robotically guided trajectory systems have been developed. Independent of technique, screw placement accuracy is paramount to achieving surgical success without the morbidity of misplaced screws. Medial breaches can lead to a neurologic deficit, superior, and inferior misplacements can injure nerve roots, and anterolateral perforations can potentially

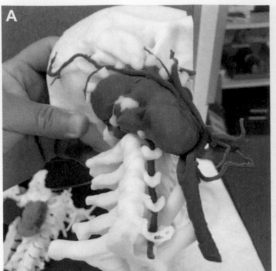
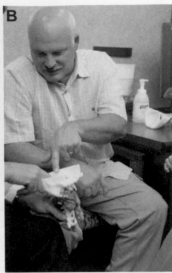

Fig. 9. Improved patient education and informed consent. (*A*) Large paraganglioma extending intracranially, involving C1–C3, causing compressive myelopathy, encasing the vertebral artery, and displacing the carotid artery. (*B*) The patient can discuss the risks, benefits, and potential morbidities with their surgeon using the patient's own anatomy and pathology to improve understanding as opposed to cross-sectional imaging and generic anatomic models.

cause vascular and visceral injuries (ie, aorta, major vessels, esophagus, and trachea).[72]

3D-printed patient-specific pedicle screw trajectory guides began to appear in the 1990s and early 2000s because of the convergence of several technologies.[73,76] To create 3DP screw guides, a preoperative 3D CT scan of the spine must be obtained. Next, a 3D model is generated as described above, and the optimal screw trajectory and size can be determined, often in consultation with the surgeon. Finally, a navigational template is designed and built with an optimal screw trajectory, the surface of which is the inverse of the posterior vertebral surface, to ensure a good fit and accuracy of screw insertion (Fig. 10). Several benefits have been shown in prospective and randomized studies, including reduced operative time, reduced blood loss, reduced intraprocedural radiation, steepening the learning curve, and, most importantly, improved pedicle screw placement accuracy.[77–85] This is particularly true in the cervical spine, in patients with complex deformities, revision surgeries, or in patients with altered anatomy secondary to tumor involvement. Although CT navigation systems have been reported to have the highest accuracy,[86] there are some drawbacks, including cost, operation complexity, increased operative times, long learning curves, and the use of ionizing radiation. Given the increasing beneficial evidence of patient matched 3D-printed guides, 2 companies, Mighty Oak

Medical (Englewood, Colorado) and Medacta MySpine TM (Castel San Pietro, Switzerland), were created to provide these services in the market for surgeons who lack a centralized POCM facility to perform VSP and manufacture of the sterilizable guides. 3D-printed guides can offer an alternative as a simple, convenient, low cost, and complex-equipment free way to improve the accuracy of pedicle screw placement.

Three-Dimensional Printed Custom Osteotomy Guides

Resection of bone tumors within the spine and sacrum can result in high complication rates and increased local recurrence rates[87] because of the complex three-dimensional geometry, limiting working corridors, and critical anatomic relationships to the spinal cord, exiting nerves, and neurovascular structures. Accurate resections with wide margins are required because this technique is associated with the lowest local recurrence rates.[88–91] Intraoperative navigation systems have been shown to improve resections by a wide margin[92,93] but they have similar limitations as described above. Patient-specific 3D-printed custom osteotomy guides, also known as patient-specific instruments (PSI), combined with VSP have allowed improved resections with negative margins, limiting the amount of bone removed.[94–99] When performed at the point of

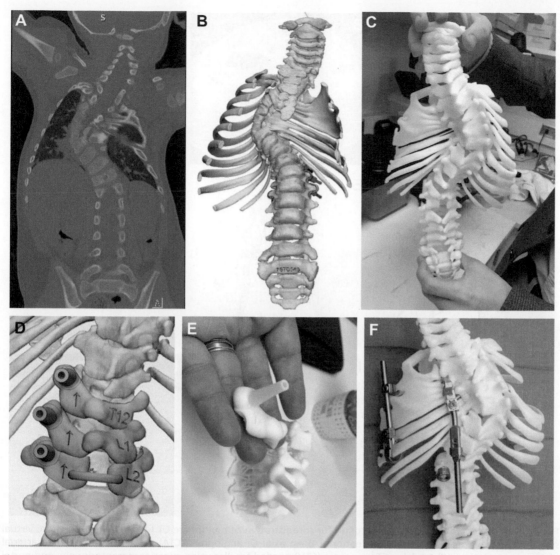

Fig. 10. 3D-printed pedicle screw trajectory guides. (*A*) Coronal CT scan demonstrating a complex congenital scoliosis in a 4 year old boy with several fused ribs. (*B*) 3D CAD model from segmentation. (*C*) Life size 3D-printed model drives further understanding to help define what the surgical plan can be. (*D*) After consultation with the model, the surgeon decided to place 3 pedicle screws at T12, L1, and L2. Pedicle screw trajectory guides were designed to subtract the underlying bone and avoid the superior and inferior facet joints, which could fuse if manipulated at this age. (*E*) 3D-printed guides using vat photopolymerization with 3D-printed fit test lamina and spinous process. (*F*) 3D-printed model was used for patient-specific surgical rehearsal and prebending the devices.

care, tumor segmentation and added margins are improved because of the inclusion of a subspecialty radiologist and the coregistration of custom multiphase CT protocols with MRI (Fig. 11). This gold standard truth can then be used to design cutting planes that limit the amount of bone to be removed and, if possible, save critical neurovascular structures. From these cutting planes, placed by the surgeon, a patient-specific 3D-printed cutting guide matched precisely to the contours of the bone is designed by an engineer within medical CAD software. Cutting guides can be designed in 2 ways. One allows the oscillating saw to fit inside a guided slot or is alternatively designed with flat edges to guide the saw along the edge of the guide (Fig. 12). The guides are then 3D-printed with biocompatible resins or polyamides such as Nylon 11 or 12.[100] Patient matched 3D-printed guides should be considered in complex resections where local control is the goal, because they provide greater safety and accuracy, improved intraoperative confidence, maintain controlled distances

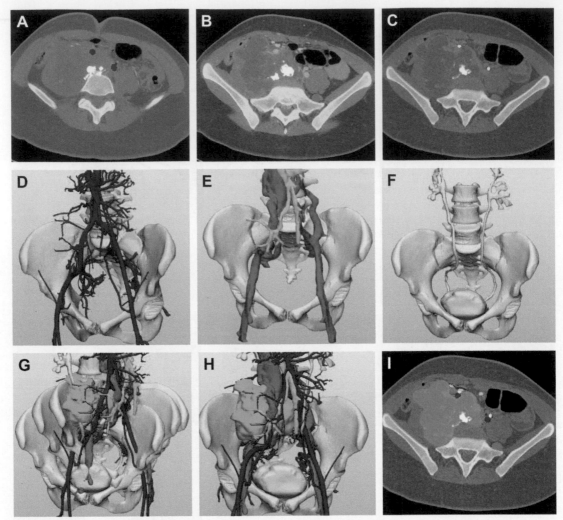

Fig. 11. Importance of radiology protocoling for coregistration of multiphase CT for oncologic resection, virtual surgical planning, and custom guide creation. (*A*) An axial CT angiogram (CTA) needed for bones and arterial phase segmentation. (*B*) 1st delay CT venogram (CTV) needed for iliac veins, superior mesenteric vein, and portal venous tributary segmentation. (*C*) CT urogram (CTU) is performed at 3 minutes and 10 minute delay for segmentation or ureteral system and bladder. (*D*) CAD representation of the arterial system and bones. (*E*) CAD representation of the venous system. Bones are segmented for coregistration. (*F*) CAD representation of the urinary collecting system. Bones are segmented for coregistration. (*G*) When the 3D CAD files are superimposed, it is clear that the patient moved between scans and in need of coregistration. (*H*) Using the N-point registration tool in 3-Matic (Materialise, Leuven, Belgium), all CAD files are co-registered to the arterial phase. (*I*) A composite mask is then made from the 3D file using Mimics software to assure that no modifications (Materialise, Leuven, Belgium) changed the position of the underlying anatomy or pathology and that the contours are accurate.

to vital structures, ability to plan and manufacture custom implants or guided allograft reconstructions, and most importantly provide tumor free margins.

THREE-DIMENSIONAL PRINTED IMPLANTS
Off the Shelf Implants: Interbody Spacers

3D printing, as an additive manufacturing technology, has allowed the design and

manufacturing of porous and mechanically proficient titanium (Ti6–Al4–V) interbody cages that mimic the porosity and stability of the native bone.[52,101–104] Given these properties, the design can enhance the delivery of osteoinductive compounds, potentially improve bone ingrowth at the fusion site,[105] and reduce stress shielding and subsidence.[106] A wide range of powder-based 3D printing techniques have been used to manufacture interbody cages for the spine via powder-

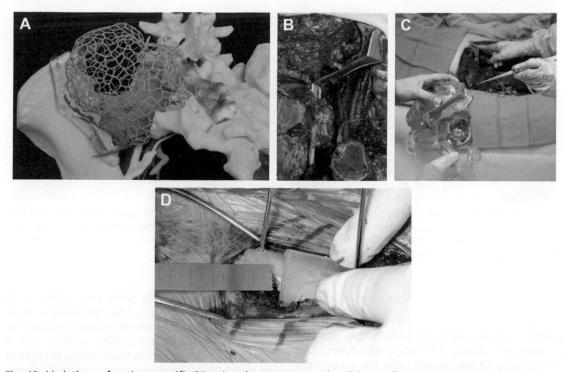

Fig. 12. Variations of patient-specific 3D-printed osteotomy guides. (*A*) Two flat edge 3D-printed guides using biocompatible resin and vat photopolymerization are designed to subtract the underlying bone with screw casings to affix to the bone. The oscillating saw is guided along the edge of the guide (*B*). Custom metal flat edges guided to perform accurate osteotomies through the iliac wing, which has already been removed. (*C*) Intraoperative use of a nonsterile model brought adjacent to the surgical field to provide the forest view and further assure accuracy. (*D*) 3D-printed osteotomy guide with slot designed for an oscillating saw to be placed, assuring the appropriate plane is followed for cutting bone at angles not perpendicular to the saw.

based printing (SLS, SLM, EBM, and DMLS). Because the benefits of 3D-printed interbody cages have been widely accepted, most major spine medical device companies now have a device commercially available as an off the shelf product, including Medtronic (Dublin, Ireland), Nuvasive (San Diego, California), Stryker (Kalamazoo, Michigan), Depuy Synthese (Raynham, Massachusetts), and Captiva Spine (Jupiter, Florida) (Fig. 13).

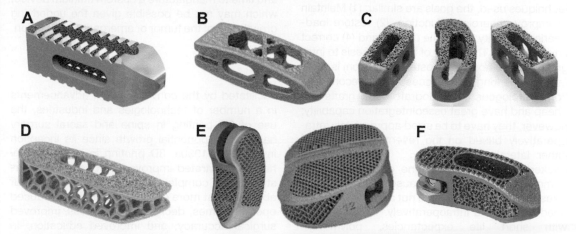

Fig. 13. 3D-printed titanium off the shelf interbody spine spacers available commercially. (*A*) Stryker tritanium PL cage. (*B*) Medtronic Adaptix cage. (*C*) Captiva Tirbolox-I titanium lumbar cage. (*D*) Nuvasive modulus XLIF cage. (*E*) Depuy Synthes Conduit Cage. (*F*) Globus Medical Hedron T Cage.

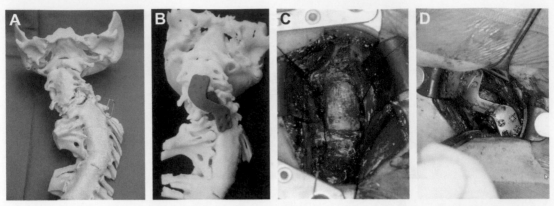

Fig. 14. 3D-printed custom titanium plate. (A) 3D-printed complex fusion and scoliosis deformity. (B) After VSP, including custom osteotomy, allograft planning, and designing a custom plate, a prototype of the reconstruction was printed for evaluation. (C) Intraoperative view after osteotomy and allograft placement were performed. (D) A custom titanium 3D-printed plate in place.

Custom Three-Dimensional Printed Implants for the Spine and Sacrum

Because of the ability to manufacture complex custom geometries and lattice structures, vary the porosity of the implant, vary the percentage of titanium versus osteoconductive materials, and produce one of a kind rapid prototypes, 3D printing is uniquely suited to make custom implants in the spine and sacrum when performing oncologic resections (Fig. 14). En bloc resections aim to remove the tumor with a margin, if possible, for aggressive benign diseases (Enneking stage 3) such as a giant cell tumor,[107] osteoblastoma,[108] or aggressive malignant disease, and primary bone tumors.[109–111] Many reconstruction techniques have been described, each with its own advantages and disadvantages, which are beyond the scope of this article. Despite the reconstruction techniques used, the goals are similar: (1) Maintain or improve neurologic function, (2) restore load-bearing capacity, (3) fill the defect, and (4) correct any deformity. The ability of the prosthesis to integrate with the host bone (osteointegration) is a key factor in the long-term success of the reconstruction. Autologous and allograft bone grafts are cheap and have great osseointegration capability; however, they have to be sized appropriately intraoperatively based on the resection and fixated either laterally or anteriorly.[112,113] Mesh cages packed with cancellous bone graft are another common technique, but because patient matched sizes without 3D printing are not available, they too need to be sized intraoperatively.[114] For patients with short life expectancies, polymethylmethacrylate shaped to the defect can be used, but it does not have osseous integration properties.[115,116] Given the complexities and unique patient-specific defects when performing single and multilevel vertebrectomies, sacrectomy, or internal and external hemipelvectomy procedures using VSP, 3D-printed cutting guides, and a customized implant, it has the potential to improve fit, distribute loads, and increase osseous integration. This is particularly true in the cervical and thoracic spines and the craniocervical junction.[117–119]

There are drawbacks, however, because it requires the surgeon to carefully follow the preoperative plan to avoid a mismatch between the resected specimen and the implant. There can be unpredictable situations that may arise intraoperatively that complicate the reconstruction, requiring traditional backup options to be available, leaving an expensive custom-manufactured device unused. Additional limitations are the cost and time to manufacture a custom titanium device, which may not be possible given the underlying growth rate of the tumor or emergent presentation.

SUMMARY

Facilitated by the convergence of advancements in a number of technologies and industries, the use of 3D printing in spine and sacral surgery has seen exponential growth since its inception in the early 1990s. 3D printing in spine surgery has demonstrated improved preoperative understanding of complex pathologies, increased our ability to treat more complex deformities, reduced operative times, decreased blood loss, improved surgical accuracy, and improved education. In addition, the ability to create patient-specific pedicle screw trajectory guides, custom osteotomy guides, and 3D-printed titanium implants has led to better clinical outcomes and reduced complications. These technologies allow personalized design, custom manufacturing, and surgeries tailored to each patient's specific needs. As 3D printing technology continues to evolve, we can expect to see further advancements in spinal and sacral surgery, improving patient outcomes and quality of life.

CLINCAL CARE POINTS

- Surgical treatment of primary and metastatic tumors involving the spine and sacrum is complex requiring a multidisciplinary team.

- 3D printing and virtual surgical planning at the point of care for patient specific life size anatomic models and 3D printed surgical guides has several advantages.

- Incorporating Engineers, 3D printers, Radiologist, and technologist into the multidisciplinary care team improves outcomes and can reduce operative times.

- 3D printing for spine and sacral tumors improves preoperative understanding and surgical planning though haptic perception and synthesizing what can be >10,000 images of CT MRI and PET Data into a single model.

- 3D printed models improve patient education and implicit trust with surgeon.

- Subspecialty radiologist segmentation of tumors provides the most accurate tumor margin necessary for long term survival.

DISCLOSURE

The authors have nothing to disclose.

REFERENCES

1. ASTM. Standard technology for additive manufacturing-General principles/Terminology. West Conshohocken (PA): ASTM ISO/ASTM 52900:2015 (E); 2015.

2. U.S. Food and Drug Administration. Technical Considerations for Additive Manufactured Medical Devices: Guidance for Industry and Food and Drug Administration Staff. 2017 Available at: https://www.fda.gov/regulatory-information/search-fda-guidance-documents/technical-considerations-additive-manufactured-medical-devices. Accessed March 29, 2022.

3. Mitsouras D, Liacouras P, Imanzadeh A, et al. Medical 3D Printing for the Radiologist. Radiographics 2015;35(07):1965–88.

4. Chen J, Bokacheva L, Rusinek H. Chapter 3: Image Segmentation and Nonuniformity Correction Methods. In: Wake N, editor. 3D printing for the radiologist. Missouri: Elsevier; 2022. p. 31–43.

5. Suetens P, Bellon E, Vandermeulen D, et al. Image segmentation: methods and applications in diagnostic radiology and nuclear medicine. Eur J Radiol 1993;17(01):14–21.

6. Wallner J, Hochegger K, Chen X, et al. Clinical evaluation of semi-automatic open-source algorithmic software segmentation of the mandibular bone: Practical feasibility and assessment of a new course of action. PLoS One 2018;13(05):e0196378.

7. Qiu B, Guo J, Kraeima J, et al. Automatic segmentation of the mandible from computed tomography scans for 3D virtual surgical planning using the convolutional neural network. Phys Med Biol 2019;64(17):175020.

8. Kraeima J, Dorgelo B, Gulbitti HA, et al. Multi-modality 3D mandibular resection planning in head and neck cancer using CT and MRI data fusion: A clinical series. Oral Oncol 2018;81:22–8.

9. Huff TJ, Ludwig PE, Zuniga JM. The potential for machine learning algorithms to improve and reduce the cost of 3-dimensional printing for surgical planning. Expert Rev Med Devices 2018; 15(05):349–56.

10. Gietema HA, Wang Y, Xu D, et al. Pulmonary nodules detected at lung cancer screening: interobserver variability of semiautomated volume measurements. Radiology 2006;241(01):251–7.

11. Wormanns D, Kohl G, Klotz E, et al. Volumetric measurements of pulmonary nodules at multi-row detector CT: in vivo reproducibility. Eur Radiol 2004;14(01):86–92.

12. Zheng B, Swensson RG, Golla S, et al. Detection and classification performance levels of mammographic masses under different computer-aided detection cueing environments. Acad Radiol 2004;11(04):398–406.

13. Qiu B, van der Wel H, Kraeima J, et al. Automatic Segmentation of Mandible from Conventional Methods to Deep Learning-A Review. J Pers Med 2021;11(07):629.

14. Cardenas CE, Yang J, Anderson BM, et al. Advances in Auto-Segmentation. Semin Radiat Oncol 2019;29(03):185–97.

15. Sears VA, Morris JM. Establishing a Point-of-Care Virtual Planning and 3D Printing Program. Semin Plast Surg 2022;36(3):133–48.

16. Sharma N, Aggarwal LM. Automated medical image segmentation techniques. J Med Phys 2010; 35(01):3–14.

17. Kamio T, Suzuki M, Asaumi R, et al. DICOM segmentation and STL creation for 3D printing: a process and software package comparison for osseous anatomy. 3D Print Med. 2020;6(01):17.

18. Kelly R, Chakravorty D. The Most Common 3D File Formats in 2022. Available at: https://all3dp.com/2/most-common-3d-file-formats-model/. Accessed March 20, 2022.

19. Christensen A, Rybicki FJ. Maintaining safety and efficacy for 3D printing in medicine. 3D Print Med. 2017;3(01):1.

20. il C. Apparatus for Production of Three-Dimensional Objects by Stereolithography. United States patent US 4,575,330A. 1986 Available at: https://patents.google.com/patent/US4575330A/en. Accessed March 29, 2022.

21. 2. Crump SS. Apparatus and Method for Creating Three-Dimensional Objects. United States patent US 5121329A. 1989 Available at: https:patents.google.com/patent/US5121329. Accessed March 29, 2022.

22. Davim JP. Additive and subtractive manufacturing: emergent technologies. Berlin: De Gruyter; 2020.

23. Liacouras P, Wake N. Chapter 5: 3D Printing Principles and Technologies. In: Wake N, editor. 3D printing for the radiologist. Missouri: Elsevier; 2022. p. 61–73.

24. Alexander AE, Wake N. Chapter 6: 3D Printed Anatomic Models and Guides. In: Wake N, editor. 3D printing for the radiologist. Missouri: Elsevier; 2022. p. 75–88.

25. Bastawrous S, Wu L, Strzelecki B, et al. Establishing Quality and Safety in Hospital-based 3D Printing Programs: Patient-first Approach. Radiographics 2021; 41(04):1208–29.

26. Liu X, Han C, Cui Y, et al. Detection and Segmentation of Pelvic Bones Metastases in MRI Images for Patients With Prostate Cancer Based on Deep Learning. Front Oncol 2021;11:773299.

27. von Schacky CE, Wilhelm NJ, Schäfer VS, et al. Multitask Deep Learning for Segmentation and Classification of Primary Bone Tumors on Radiographs. Radiology 2021;301(2):398–406.

28. Liu X, Han C, Wang H, et al. Fully automated pelvic bone segmentation in multiparameteric MRI using a 3D convolutional neural network. Insights Imaging 2021;12(1):93.

29. Bloem JL, Reidsma II. Bone and soft tissue tumors of hip and pelvis. Eur J Radiol 2012;81(12): 3793–801.

30. Calhoun PS, Kuszyk BS, Heath DG, et al. Three-dimensional volume rendering of spiral CT data: theory and method. Radiographics 1999;19:745–64.

31. Li AE, Fishman EK. Cervical spine trauma: evaluation by multidetector CT and three-dimensional volume rendering. Emerg Radiol 2003;10:34–9.

32. Salvolini L, Bichi Secchi E, et al. Clinical applications of 2D and 3D CT imaging of the airways: a review. Eur J Radiol 2000;34:9–25.

33. Fox LA, Vannier MW, West OC, et al. Diagnostic performance of CT, MPR and 3DCT imaging in maxillofacial trauma. Comput Med Imaging Graph 1995;19:385–95.

34. Pretorius ES, Fishman EK. Spiral CT and Three Dimensional CT of Musculoskeletal Pathology. Radiol Clin North Am 1999;37:953–74.

35. Wu B, Klatzky RL, Stetten G. Visualizing 3D objects from 2D cross sectional images displayed in-situ versus ex-situ. J Exp Psychol Appl 2010;16(1):45–59.

36. National Research Council. Learning to Think spatially. Washington, DC: National Academies Press; 2006.

37. Hegarty M, Keehner M, Cohen C, et al. The role of spatial cognition in medicine: Applications for selecting and training professionals. Applied Spatial Cognition 2007;285–315.

38. Heinrich H, Bülthoff SY, et al. How Are Three-Dimensional Objects Represented in the Brain? Cerebr Cortex 1995;5(3):247–60.

39. McDonald RJ, Schwartz KM, Eckel LJ, et al. The effects of changes in utilization and technological advancements of cross-sectional imaging on radiologist workload. Acad Radiol 2015;22(9):1191–8.

40. Izatt MT, Thorpe PL, Thompson RG, et al. The use of physical biomodelling in complex spinal surgery. Eur Spine J 2007;16(9):1507–18.

41. D'Urso PS, Askin GN, Earwaker WJS, et al. Spinal biomodeling. Spine 1999;24(12):1247–51.

42. Zheng B, Wang X, Zheng Y, et al. 3D-printed model improves clinical assessment of surgeons on anatomy. J Robot Surg 2019;13(1):61–7.

43. Chepelev L, Wake N, Ryan J, et al. RSNA Special Interest Group for 3D Printing. Radiological Society of North America (RSNA) 3D printing Special Interest Group (SIG): guidelines for medical 3D printing and appropriateness for clinical scenarios. 3D Print Med. 2018;4(1):11.

44. Amendola L, Cappuccio M, De lure F, et al. En bloc resections for primary spinal tumors in 20 years of experience: effectiveness and safety. Spine J 2014;14:2608–17.

45. Boriani S, De lure F, Bandiera S, et al. Chondrosarcoma of the mobile spine: report on 22 cases. Spine 2000;25:804–12.

46. Boriani S, Bandiera S, Biagini R, et al. Chordoma of the mobile spine: fifty years of experience. Spine 2006;31:493–503.

47. Boriani S, Bandiera S, Casadei R, et al. Giant cell tumor of the mobile spine. A review of 49 cases. Spine 2012;37:E37–45.

48. Cohen ZR, Fourney DR, Marco RA, et al. Total cervical spondylectomy for primary osteogenic sarcoma. Case report and description of operative technique. J Neurosurg 2002;97(3 Suppl):386–92.

49. Yamazaki T, McLoughlin GS, Patel S, et al. Feasibility and safety of en bloc resection for primary spine tumors: a systematic review by the Spine Oncology Study Group. Spine 2009;34(22 Suppl): S31–8.

50. Currier BL, Papagelopoulos PJ, Krauss WE, et al. Total en bloc spondylectomy of C5 vertebra for chordoma. Spine 2007;32:E294–9.

51. Xiao JR, Huang WD, Yang XH, et al. En Bloc Resection of Primary Malignant Bone Tumor in the Cervical Spine Based on 3-Dimensional Printing Technology. Orthop Surg 2016;8(2):171–8.

52. Choy WJ, Parr WCH, Phan K, et al. 3-dimensional printing for anterior cervical surgery: a review. J Spine Surg 2018;4(4):757–69.

53. Wilcox B, Mobbs RJ, Wu AM, et al. Systematic review of 3D printing in spinal surgery: the current state of play. J Spine Surg 2017;3(3):433–43.

54. Guarino J, Tennyson S, McCain G, et al. Rapid prototyping technology for surgeries of the pediatric spine and pelvis: benefits analysis. J Pediatr Orthop 2007;27:955–60.

55. Wang YT, Yang XJ, Yan B, et al. Clinical application of three-dimensional printing in the personalized treatment of complex spinal disorders. Chin J Traumatol 2016;19:31–4.

56. Leary OP, Crozier J, Liu DD, et al. Three-Dimensional Printed Anatomic Modeling for Surgical Planning and Real-Time Operative Guidance in Complex Primary Spinal Column Tumors: Single-Center Experience and Case Series. World Neurosurg 2021;145:e116–26.

57. Ozturk AM, Sirinturk S, Kucuk L, et al. Multidisciplinary Assessment of Planning and Resection of Complex Bone Tumor Using Patient-Specific 3D Model. Indian J Surg Oncol 2019;10(1):115–24.

58. Lador R, Regev G, Salame K, et al. Use of 3-Dimensional Printing Technology in Complex Spine Surgeries. World Neurosurg 2020;133:e327–41.

59. Liew Y, Beveridge E, Demetriades AK, et al. 3D printing of patient-specific anatomy: A tool to improve patient consent and enhance imaging interpretation by trainees. Br J Neurosurg 2015; 29:712–4.

60. Hu P, Sun J, Wei F, et al. Patient-Tailored 3D-Printing Models in the Subspecialty Training of Spinal Tumors: A Comparative Study and Questionnaire Survey. World Neurosurg 2022;161:e488–94.

61. Blohm JE, Salinas PA, Avila MJ, et al. Three-Dimensional Printing in Neurosurgery Residency Training: A Systematic Review of the Literature. World Neurosurg 2022;161:111–22.

62. Lederman SJ, Klatzky RL. Haptic perception: a tutorial. Atten Percept Psychophys 2009;71(7): 1439–60.

63. Matsumoto J, Wang K. Chapter 8: Documentation and Reimbursement for 3D Printed Anatomic Models and Guides. In: Wake N, editor. 3D printing for the radiologist. Missouri: Elsevier; 2022. p. 99–108.

64. American Medical Association. September 2018 CPT Editorial summary of Panel Actions. 2018 Available at: https://www.ama-assn.org/system/

files/2018-10/september-2018-summary-panel-actions.pdf. Accessed March 11, 2022.

65. American Society of Mechanical Engineers (ASME). 3D Printing at the Point of Care. Available at: https://resources.asme.org/poc3dp-events. Accessed December 14, 2021.

66. Parker SL, McGirt MJ, Farber SH, et al. Accuracy of free-hand pedicle screws in the thoracic and lumbar spine: analysis of 6816 consecutive screws. Neurosurgery 2011;68(1):170–8.

67. Holly LT, Foley KT. Three-dimensional fluoroscopy-guided percutaneous thoracolumbar pedicle screw placement. Technical note. J Neurosurg 2003;99(3 suppl):324–9.

68. Youkilis AS, Quint DJ, McGillicuddy JE, et al. Stereotactic navigation for placement of pedicle screws in the thoracic spine. Neurosurgery 2001; 48(4):771–8.

69. Fu TS, Chen LH, Wong CB, et al. Computer-assisted fluoroscopic navigation of pedicle screw insertion: an in vivo feasibility study. Acta Orthop Scand 2004;75(6):730–5.

70. Amiot LP, Lang K, Putzier M, et al. Comparative results between conventional and computer-assisted pedicle screw installation in the thoracic, lumbar, and sacral spine. Spine 2000;25(5):606–14.

71. Sarwahi V, Wendolowski SF, Gecelter RC, et al. Are We Underestimating the Significance of Pedicle Screw Misplacement? Spine 2016;41(9):E548–55.

72. Goffin J, Van Brussel K, Vander Sloten J, et al. 3D-CT based, personalized drill guide for posterior transarticular screw fixation at C1–C2: technical note. Neuro Orthoped 1999;25:47–56.

73. Goffin J, Van Brussel K, Martens K, et al. Three-dimensional computed tomography-based, personalized drill guide for posterior cervical stabilization at C1–C2. Spine 2001;26(12):1343–7.

74. Ryken TC, Owen BD, Christensen GE, et al. Image-based drill templates for cervical pedicle screw placement. J Neurosurg Spine 2009 Jan;10(1): 21–6.

75. Sugawara T, Higashiyama N, Kaneyama S, et al. Multistep pedicle screw insertion procedure with patient-specific lamina fit-and-lock templates for the thoracic spine: clinical article. J Neurosurg Spine 2013;19(2):185–90.

76. Sugawara T, Kaneyama S, Higashiyama N, et al. Prospective multicenter study of a multistep screw insertion technique using patient-specific screw guide templates for the cervical and thoracic spine. Spine 2018;43(23):1685–94.

77. Fan Y, Du JP, Wu QN, et al. Accuracy of a patient-specific template for pedicle screw placement compared with a conventional method: a meta-analysis. Arch Orthop Trauma Surg 2017;137(12): 1641–9.

78. Bundoc RC, Delgado GG, Grozman SA. A novel patient-specific drill guide template for pedicle screw insertion into the subaxial cervical spine utilizing stereolithographic modelling: an in vitro study. Asian Spine J 2017;11(1):4–14.

79. Cecchinato R, Berjano P, Zerbi A, et al. Pedicle screw insertion with patient-specific 3D-printed guides based on low-dose CT scan is more accurate than free-hand technique in spine deformity patients: a prospective, randomized clinical trial. Eur Spine J 2019;28(7):1712–23.

80. Cool J, van Schuppen J, de Boer MA, et al. Accuracy assessment of pedicle screw insertion with patient specific 3D-printed guides through superimpose CT-analysis in thoracolumbar spinal deformity surgery. Eur Spine J 2021;30(11):3216–24.

81. Garg B, Gupta M, Singh M, et al. Outcome and safety analysis of 3D-printed patient-specific pedicle screw jigs for complex spinal deformities: a comparative study. Spine J 2019;19(1):56–64.

82. Pijpker PAJ, Kraeima J, Witjes MJH, et al. Accuracy of Patient-Specific 3D-Printed Drill Guides for Pedicle and Lateral Mass Screw Insertion: An Analysis of 76 Cervical and Thoracic Screw Trajectories. Spine 2021;46(3):160–8.

83. Li Y, Lin J, Wang Y, et al. Comparative study of 3D printed navigation template-assisted atlantoaxial pedicle screws versus free-hand screws for type II odontoid fractures. Eur Spine J 2021;30:498–506.

84. Liang W, Han B, Hai JJ, et al. 3D-printed drill guide template, a promising tool to improve pedicle screw placement accuracy in spinal deformity surgery: A systematic review and meta-analysis. Eur Spine J 2021;30:1173–83.

85. Meng M, Wang J, Sun T, et al. Clinical applications and prospects of 3D printing guide templates in orthopaedics. J Orthop Translat 2022;34:22–41.

86. Perdomo-Pantoja A, Ishida W, Zygourakis C, et al. Accuracy of Current Techniques for Placement of Pedicle Screws in the Spine: A Comprehensive Systematic Review and Meta-Analysis of 51,161 Screws. World Neurosurg 2019;126:664–78.

87. Delloye C, Banse X, Brichard B, et al. Pelvic reconstruction with a structural pelvic allograft after resection of a malignant bone tumor. J Bone Joint Surg 2007;89(3):579–87.

88. Han I, Lee YM, Cho HS, et al. Outcome after surgical treatment of pelvic sarcomas. Clin Orthop Surg 2010;2(3):160–6.

89. Ozaki T, Flege S, Kevric M, et al. Osteosarcoma of the pelvis: experience of the Cooperative Osteosarcoma Study Group. J Clin Oncol 2003;21(2):334–41.

90. Hoffmann C, Ahrens S, Dunst J, et al. Pelvic Ewing sarcoma: a retrospective analysis of 241 cases. Cancer 1999;85(4):869–77.

91. Sluga M, Windhager R, Lang S, et al. The role of surgery and resection margins in the treatment of Ewing's sarcoma. Clin Orthop Relat Res 2001;(392):394–9.

92. Jeys L, Matharu GS, Nandra RS, et al. Can computer navigation-assisted surgery reduce the risk of an intralesional margin and reduce the rate of local recurrence in patients with a tumour of the pelvis or sacrum? Bone and Joint Journal 2013;95(10):1417–24.

93. So TYC, Lam YL, Mak KL. Computer-assisted navigation in bone tumor surgery: seamless workflow model and evolution of technique. Clin Orthop Relat Res 2010;468(11):2985–91.

94. Gouin F, Paul L, Odri GA, et al. Computer-Assisted Planning and Patient-Specific Instruments for Bone Tumor Resection within the Pelvis: A Series of 11 Patients. Sarcoma 2014;2014:842709.

95. Khan FA, Lipman JD, Pearle AD, et al. Surgical technique: computer-generated custom jigs improve accuracy of wide resection of bone tumors. Clin Orthop Relat Res 2013;471:2007–16.

96. Jentzsch T, Vlachopoulos L, Fürnstahl P, et al. Tumor resection at the pelvis using three-dimensional planning and patient-specific instruments: a case series. World J Surg Oncol 2016;14(1):249.

97. Cartiaux O, Paul L, Francq BG, et al. Improved accuracy with 3D planning and patient-specific instruments during simulated pelvic bone tumor surgery. Ann Biomed Eng 2014;42(1):205–13.

98. Biscaccianti V, Fragnaud H, Hascoët JY, et al. Digital chain for pelvic tumor resection with 3D-printed surgical cutting guides. Front Bioeng Biotechnol 2022;10:991676.

99. Evrard R, Schubert T, Paul L, et al. Resection margins obtained with patient-specific instruments for resecting primary pelvic bone sarcomas: A case-control study. Orthop Traumatol Surg Res 2019;105(4):781–7.

100. International Organization for Standardization. Standard 10993:2009: Biological evaluation of medical devices. 4th edition. Geneva (Switzerland): International Organization for Standardization; 2009.

101. Hollander DA, von Walter M, Wirtz T, et al. Structural, mechanical and in vitro characterization of individually structured Ti-6Al-4V produced by direct laser forming. Biomaterials 2006;27(7):955–63.

102. Seaman S, Kerezoudis P, Bydon M, et al. Titanium vs. polyetheretherketone (PEEK) interbody fusion: Meta-analysis and review of the literature. J Clin Neurosci 2017;44:23–9.

103. Lin CY, Wirtz T, LaMarca F, et al. Structural and mechanical evaluations of a topology optimized titanium interbody fusion cage fabricated by selective laser melting process. J Biomed Mater Res 2007;83(2):272–9.

104. Serra T, Capelli C, Toumpaniari R, et al. Design and fabrication of 3D-printed anatomically shaped lumbar cage for intervertebral disc (IVD) degeneration treatment. Biofabrication 2016;8(3):035001.

105. Adl Amini D, Moser M, Oezel L, et al. Fusion assessment in standalone lateral lumbar interbody fusion: 3D-printed titanium versus polyetheretherketone (PEEK) cages. J Spine Surg 2022;8(3): 323–32.

106. Provaggi E, Leong JJH, Kalaskar DM. Applications of 3D printing in the management of severe spinal conditions. Proc Inst Mech Eng H 2017;231(6): 471–86.

107. Charest-Morin R, Fisher CG, Varga PP, et al. En bloc resection versus intralesional surgery in the treatment of giant cell tumor of the spine. Spine 2017;42(18):1383–90.

108. Versteeg AL, Dea N, Boriani S, et al. Surgical management of spinal osteoblastomas. J Neurosurg Spine 2017;7:1–7.

109. Dekutoski MB, Clarke MJ, Rose P, et al. (2016) Osteosarcoma of the spine: prognostic variables for local recurrence and overall survival, a multicenter ambispective study. J Neurosurg Spine 2017; 25(1):59–68.

110. Fisher CG, Versteeg AL, Dea N, et al. Surgical management of spinal chondrosarcomas. Spine 2016;41(8):678–85.

111. Gokaslan ZL, Zadnik PL, Sciubba DM, et al. Mobile spine chordoma: results of 166 patients from the AOSpine Knowledge Forum Tumor database. J Neurosurg Spine 2016;24(4):644–51.

112. Vaz K, Verma K, Protopsaltis T, et al. Bone grafting options for lumbar spine surgery: a review examining clinical efficacy and complications. SAS J 2010;4(3):75–86.

113. Oppenlander ME, Maulucci CM, Ghobrial GM, et al. En Bloc Resection of Upper Thoracic Chordoma via a Combined Simultaneous Anterolateral Thoracoscopic and Posterior Approach. Operative Neurosurgery 2014;10(3):380–6.

114. Dang L, Liu Z, Liu X, et al. Sagittal en bloc resection of primary tumors in the thoracic and lumbar spine: feasibility, safety and outcome. Sci Rep 2020;10(1): 9108.

115. Fourney DR, Abi-Said D, Rhines LD, et al. Simultaneous anterior-posterior approach to the thoracic and lumbar spine for the radical resection of tumors followed by reconstruction and stabilization. J Neurosurg 2001;94(2 Suppl):232–44.

116. Salem KM, Fisher CG. Anterior column reconstruction with PMMA: an effective long-term alternative in spinal oncologic surgery. Eur Spine J 2016; 25(12):3916–22.

117. Xu N, Wei F, Liu X, et al. Reconstruction of the Upper Cervical Spine Using a Personalized 3D-Printed Vertebral Body in an Adolescent With Ewing Sarcoma. Spine 2016;41(1):E50.

118. Choy WJ, Mobbs RJ, Wilcox B, et al. Reconstruction of Thoracic Spine Using a Personalized 3D-Printed Vertebral Body in Adolescent with T9 Primary Bone Tumor. World Neurosurg 2017;105. 1032.e13-17.

119. Girolami M, Boriani S, Bandiera S, et al. Biomimetic 3D-printed custom-made prosthesis for anterior column reconstruction in the thoracolumbar spine: a tailored option following en bloc resection for spinal tumors : Preliminary results on a case-series of 13 patients. Eur Spine J 2018;27(12):3073–83.

Moving?

Make sure your subscription moves with you!

To notify us of your new address, find your **Clinics Account Number** (located on your mailing label above your name), and contact customer service at:

Email: journalscustomerservice-usa@elsevier.com

800-654-2452 (subscribers in the U.S. & Canada)
314-447-8871 (subscribers outside of the U.S. & Canada)

Fax number: 314-447-8029

Elsevier Health Sciences Division
Subscription Customer Service
3251 Riverport Lane
Maryland Heights, MO 63043

*To ensure uninterrupted delivery of your subscription, please notify us at least 4 weeks in advance of move.

Moving?

Make sure your subscription moves with you!

To notify us of your new address, find your Clinics Account Number (located on your mailing label above your name), and contact customer service at:

Email: journalscustomerservice-usa@elsevier.com

800-654-2452 (subscribers in the U.S. & Canada)
314-447-8871 (subscribers outside of the U.S. & Canada)

Fax number 314-447-8029

Elsevier Health Sciences Division
Subscription Customer Service
3251 Riverport Lane
Maryland Heights, MO 63043

Printed and bound by CPI Group (UK) Ltd, Croydon, CR0 4YY

03/10/2024

01040367-0014